Pocket Notes for the Physical Therapist Assistant

Steven B. Skinner PT, MS, EdD

Christina Hurley PT, MA

both at
Kingsborough Community College
City University of New York
Brooklyn, New York

D1611678

JONES AND BARTLETT PUBLISHERS
Sudbury, Massachusetts
BOSTON   TORONTO   LONDON   SINGAPORE

World Headquarters

Jones and Bartlett
Publishers
40 Tall Pine Drive
Sudbury, MA 01776
978-443-5000
info@jbpub.com
www.jbpub.com

Jones and Bartlett
Publishers Canada
6339 Ormindale Way
Mississauga, ON L5V 1J2
CANADA

Jones and Bartlett
Publishers International
Barb House,
Barb Mews
London W6 7PA
UK

Jones and Bartlett's books and products are available through most book-
stores and online booksellers. To contact Jones and Bartlett Publishers directly, call 800-832-0034, fax 978-443-8000, or visit our website at
www.jbpub.com.

Substantial discounts on bulk quantities of Jones and Bartlett's publications are available to corporations, professional associations, and other
qualified organizations. For details and specific discount information,
contact the special sales department at Jones and Bartlett via the above
contact information or send an email to specialsales@jbpub.com.

ISBN-13: 978-0-7637-3811-2
ISBN-10: 0-7637-3811-5

6048

Production Credits
Executive Editor: David Cella
Editorial Assistant: Lisa Gordon
Production Director: Amy Rose
Production Editor: Renée Sekerak
Associate Marketing Manager: Laura Kavigian
Manufacturing Buyer: Amy Bacus
Composition: Paw Print Media
Cover Design: Anne Spencer
Printing and Binding: Transcontinental-Metrolitho
Cover Printing: Transcontinental-Metrolitho

Printed in Canada
10 09 08 07   10 9 8 7 6 5 4 3 2 1

Dedication

To my family, Sheila, Malcolm, and Niani, with much love.

—SBS

To my family and friends, thank you for all your love and support.

—CH

Contents

Preface

We have observed physical therapist assistant (PTA) students and new graduates struggle with the anxieties of competent clinical practice. We thought an easy "one-stop shopping" text of relevant clinical data might ease some anxiety by providing students with quick didactic support. Therefore, this book is not meant to be a primary learning source or an exhaustive treatise of physical therapy practice. Instead, it is intended to be used as a clinical reference guide: a text containing useful and easily retrievable data that supports clinical practice.

This book is organized in six chapters and an appendix of commonly used abbreviations. To facilitate easier retrieval, all data are organized in columnar or tabular form. The first chapter contains clinical assessment data including range of motion, manual muscle testing, blood values and vital signs, and other useful information. It represents a compilation of those tests and values the PTA commonly encounters, interprets, and applies.

The second chapter not only reviews the basics of selected physical therapy modalities, but also provides assessment and documentation tips. The third chapter provides descriptions and goals of common therapeutic exercises as well as suggested patient instructions. The fourth chapter reviews normal gait, describes common deviations and compensations, and provides descriptions of common prosthetic gait deviations. The fifth chapter lists and describes common intravenous and oral medications. Chapter six reviews selected common pathologies including a clinical description, physical therapy goals, clinical precautions, and effective physical therapy interventions.

CHAPTER

1

Normal Values and Assessments

ASIA Classification of Spinal Cord Injury

- The American Spinal Injury Association (ASIA) has developed a spinal injury classification system based on specific motor and sensory assessments as depicted in the figure on page 2.
- Motor function is determined by manual muscle testing of 10 key muscles. Results of manual muscle tests are expressed numerically.
- Dermatomal sensation assessment for pin prick and light touch is performed and scored numerically.
- The ASIA Impairment Scale, using letters A to E, represents the overall classification of the spinal injury.

STANDARD NEUROLOGICAL CLASSIFICATION OF SPINAL CORD INJURY

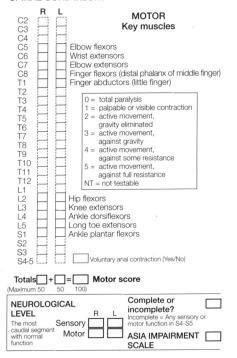

Figure 1.1   Standard Neurological Classification of Spinal Cord Injury

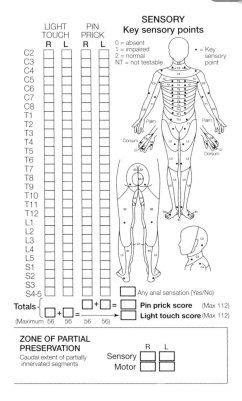

Figure 1.1   *continued*

☐ **A = Complete:** No motor or sensory function is preserved in the sacral segments S4–S5.

☐ **B = Incomplete:** Sensory but not motor function is preserved below the neurological level and includes the sacral segments S4–S5.

☐ **C = Incomplete:** Motor function is preserved below the neurological level, and more than half of key muscles below the neurological level have a muscle grade less than 3.

☐ **D = Incomplete:** Motor function is preserved below the neurological level, and at least half of key muscles below the neurological level have a muscle grade of 3 or more.

☐ **E = Normal:** motor and sensory function are normal.

Clinical Syndromes

☐ Central Cord
☐ Brown-Sequard
☐ Anterior Cord
☐ Conus Medullaris
☐ Cauda Equina

Figure 1.2   ASIA Impairment Scale

Source: Reproduced with permission of the American Spinal Injury Association (2005).

Blood—Complete Blood Count (CBC)

Note: Normal values may vary from one lab to another. The values presented in these charts should not be considered absolute.

Assessment Component	Values	Description/Implications/Red Flag Values
Red Blood Cells (RBC) (erythrocytes)	Infants: 5.5–6.0 million/mm^3 Children: 4.6–4.8 million/mm^3 Men: 4.5–5.3 million/mm^3 Women: 4.1–5.1 million/mm^3	Individuals with lower-than-normal values have anemia. Anemia symptoms: fatigue, weakness, SOB, dizziness, tachycardia Individuals with higher-than-normal values have polycythemia. Polycythemia symptoms: SOB, headache, dizziness, itchiness
Erythrocyte Sedimentation Rate (ESR/Sed. Rate)	Children: 1–13 mm/hr Men: 0–17 mm/hr Women: 1–25 mm/hr	The ESR is the rate at which erythrocytes settle out of blood plasma in 1 hour. A high rate is indicative of infection or inflammation.

continues

Blood —Complete Blood Count (CBC), cont.

Note: Normal values may vary from one lab to another. The values presented in these charts should not be considered absolute.

Assessment Component	Values	Description/Implications/Red Flag Values
Hematocrit (HCT)	Infants: 30%–60% Children: 30%–49% Men: 37%–49% Women: 36%–46%	Hematocrit is the percent of whole blood composed of erythrocytes. Exercise may be restricted at values ≤25%.
Hemoglobin (HGB)	Infants: 17–19g/dL Children: 14–17g/dL Men: 13–18g/dL Women: 12–16g/dL	HGB measures the oxygen-carrying capacity of RBCs. Low values between 8–10g/dL are associated with poor exercise tolerance, increased fatigue, and tachycardia.
Platelets	Units: cells/mm^3 Infants: 200,000–475,000	

Blood—Complete Blood Count (CBC), cont.

Note: Normal values may vary from one lab to another. The values presented in these charts should not be considered absolute.

Assessment Component	Values	Description/Implications/Red Flag Values
	Children: 150,000–400,000 Adults: 150,000–400,000	Platelets play a key role in the initiation of the clotting process within damaged blood vessels. Exercise may be cautiously performed with values of 21,000–50,000 cells/mm^3. Exercise may be contraindicated at values ≤20,000 cells/mm^3.
White Blood Cells (WBCs)	Units: cells/mm^3 Children: 4,500–14,500 Adults: 4,500–11,000	White blood cells play a crucial role in the body's immune reaction. Exercise may not be permitted at values ≤5000 cells/mm^3.
Differential WBC Count	**Neutrophils:** 1800–7000 cells/mm^3	The various white blood cells play different roles in the immune process. They exist in stereotypical proportions.

continues

Blood—Complete Blood Count (CBC), cont.

Note: Normal values may vary from one lab to another. The values presented in these charts should not be considered absolute.

Assessment Component	Values	Description/Implications/Red Flag Values
	Lymphocytes: 1500–4000 cells/mm^3 **Monocytes:** 0–800 cells/mm^3 **Eosinophils:** 0–450 cells/mm^3 **Basophils:** 0–200 cells/mm^3	

continues

Blood—Electrolytes

Note: Normal values may vary from one lab to another. The values presented in these charts should not be considered absolute.

Assessment Component	Values	Description/Implications/Red Flag Values
Potassium	Children: 3.5–5.5 mEq/L Adults: 3.5–5.3 mEq/L	Hypokalemia: dizziness, muscle weakness, fatigue, and leg cramps Hyperkalemia: muscle weakness, flaccid paralysis, paresthesias
Sodium	135–145 mEq/L	Hyponatremia: muscle twitching, weakness Hypernatremia: fever, convulsions
Chloride	Children: 98–105 mEq/L Adults: 95–105 mEq/L	Chloride shifts are most often associated with shifts in sodium.

Blood —Electrolytes, cont.

Note: Normal values may vary from one lab to another. The values presented in these charts should not be considered absolute.

Assessment Component	Values	Description/Implications/Red Flag Values
Calcium	Children: 9–11.5 mg/dL	Hypocalcemia: paresthesias, muscle spasms
	Adults: 9–11 mg/dL	Hypercalcemia: lethargy, muscle weakness, flaccidity, bone pain
Magnesium	Children: 1.6–2.6 mEq/L	Hypomagnesemia: muscle cramping, tetany, confusion
	Adults: 1.5–2.5 mEq/L	Hypermagnesemia: decreased reflexes, muscle weakness, lethargy

Blood—Prothrombin Time

Note: Normal values may vary from one lab to another. The values presented in these charts should not be considered absolute.

Assessment Component	Values	Description/Implications/Red Flag Values
Prothrombin Time (PT)	12–15 sec	This assessment measures the clotting ability of blood.
Partial Prothrombin Time (PTT)	30–40 sec	Measures 1.5 to 2.5 times the reference range are considered therapeutic. Physical therapy may be contraindicated at values ≥2.5 times the reference range in individuals not taking anticoagulants and values ≥2.5–3.0 times the reference range for those taking anticoagulant medications.

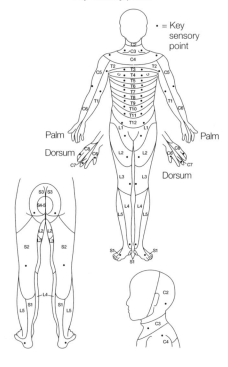

Figure 1.3   Key Sensory Points

Source: Reproduced with permission of the American Spinal Injury Association (2005).

continues

Range of Motion—Lower Extremity and Spine

Note: Values according to the American Academy of Orthopedic Surgeons.

Joint	Motion	Range of Motion (in degrees)
Hip	Flexion	0–120
	Extension	0–30
	Adduction	0–30
	Abduction	0–45
	Lateral rotation	0–45
	Medial rotation	0–45
Knee	Flexion	0–150
Ankle	Dorsiflexion	0–20
	Plantar flexion	0–50
	Inversion	0–35
	Eversion	0–15

Range of Motion—Lower Extremity and Spine, cont.

Note: Values according to the American Academy of Orthopedic Surgeons.

Spinal Segment	Motion	Range of Motion (in degrees)
Cervical	Flexion	0–45
	Extension	0–45
	Rotation	0–60
	Lateral flexion	0–45
Thoracolumbar	Flexion	0–80
	Extension	0–25
	Rotation	0–35
	Lateral flexion	0–45

Range of Motion—Lower Extremity Percentages

In some instances, it may be preferable to report measured range of motion as a percentage of normal values. This may be especially true when setting or interpreting long- and short-term goals and for reporting to third-party payers or nonphysical therapy personnel. The chart on page 16 provides percentage approximations in 5% intervals. An approximate percentage can be determined by choosing the number from the chart that is closest to the measured joint range (e.g., 95° of knee flexion represents an approximate 30% deficit).

Range of Motion—Lower Extremity Percentages

% of Normal	100	95	90	85	80	75	70	65	60	55	50	45	40	35	30	25	20	15	10	5
% Deficit	0	5	10	15	20	25	30	35	40	45	50	55	60	65	70	75	80	85	90	95
Hip flex.	120	114	108	102	96	90	84	78	72	66	60	54	48	42	36	30	24	18	12	6
Abd.	45	43	41	38	36	34	32	29	27	25	23	20	18	16	14	11	9	7	5	2
Add.	30	29	27	26	24	23	21	20	18	17	15	14	12	11	9	8	6	5	3	2
Ext. rot.	45	43	41	38	36	34	32	29	27	25	23	20	18	16	14	11	9	7	5	2
Int. rot.	45	43	41	38	36	34	32	29	27	25	23	20	18	16	14	11	9	7	5	2
Ext.	30	29	27	26	24	23	21	20	18	17	15	14	12	11	9	8	6	5	3	2
Knee flex.	135	128	122	115	108	101	95	88	81	74	68	61	54	47	41	34	27	20	14	7
Ankle dorsi.	20	19	18	17	16	15	14	13	12	11	10	9	8	7	6	5	4	3	2	1
Plantar	50	48	45	43	40	38	35	33	30	28	25	23	20	18	15	13	10	8	5	3
Invers.	35	33	32	30	28	26	25	23	21	19	18	16	14	12	11	9	7	5	4	2
Evers.	15	14	14	13	12	11	10	9	8	8	7	6	5	5	4	3	2	2	1	1

continues

Range of Motion—Upper Extremity

Note: Values according to the American Academy of Orthopedic Surgeons.

Joint	Motion	Range of Motion (in degrees)
Shoulder	Flexion	**0–180**
	Extension	**0–60**
	Abduction	**0–180**
	Lateral rotation	**0–90**
	Medial rotation	**0–70**
Elbow Complex	Flexion	**0–150**
	Pronation	**0–80**
	Supination	**0–80**
Wrist	Flexion	**0–80**
	Extension	**0–70**
	Radial deviation	**0–20**
	Ulnar deviation	**0–30**

Range of Motion—Upper Extremity, cont.

Note: Values according to the American Academy of Orthopedic Surgeons.

Joint	Motion	Range of Motion (in degrees)
Thumb	CMC flexion	0–15
	CMC extension	0–20
	CMC abduction	0–70
	MCP flexion	0–50
	IP flexion	0–80
2nd through 5th digits	MCP flexion	0–90
	MCP hyperextension	0–45
	MCP abduction	0–45
	PIP flexion	0–100
	DIP flexion	0–90
	DIP hyperextension	0–10

continues

Range of Motion—Upper Extremity Percentages

(See rationale and use instructions on page 15.)

% of Normal	100	95	90	85	80	75	70	65	60	55	50	45	40	35	30	25	20	15	10	5
% Deficit	0	5	10	15	20	25	30	35	40	45	50	55	60	65	70	75	80	85	90	95
Shld. abd.	180	171	162	153	144	135	126	117	108	99	90	81	72	63	54	45	36	27	18	9
Flexion	180	171	162	153	144	135	126	117	108	99	90	81	72	63	54	45	36	27	18	9
Ext. rot.	90	86	81	77	72	68	63	59	54	50	45	41	36	32	27	23	18	14	9	5
Int. rot.	70	67	63	60	56	53	49	46	42	39	35	32	28	25	21	18	14	11	7	4
Extension	60	57	54	51	48	45	42	39	36	33	30	27	24	21	18	15	12	9	6	3
Elbow *flex.*	150	143	135	128	120	113	105	98	90	83	75	68	60	53	45	38	30	23	15	8
Pron./Supin.	80	76	72	68	64	60	56	52	48	44	40	36	32	28	24	20	17	12	8	4
Wrist Flexion	80	76	72	68	64	60	56	52	48	44	40	36	32	28	24	20	17	12	8	4
Ext.	70	67	63	60	56	53	49	46	42	39	35	32	28	25	21	18	14	11	7	4
Rad. dev.	20	19	18	17	16	15	14	13	12	11	10	9	8	7	6	5	4	3	2	1
Uln. dev.	30	29	27	26	24	23	21	20	18	17	15	14	12	11	9	8	6	5	3	2

Range of Motion—Upper Extremity, cont.

(See rationale and use instructions on page 15.)

% of Normal	100	95	90	85	80	75	70	65	60	55	50	45	40	35	30	25	20	15	10	5
% Deficit	0	5	10	15	20	25	30	35	40	45	50	55	60	65	70	75	80	85	90	95
Thumb																				
CMC flex.	15	14	14	13	12	11	11	10	9	8	8	7	6	5	5	4	3	2	2	1
CMC ext.	20	19	18	17	16	15	14	13	12	11	10	9	8	7	6	5	4	3	2	1
CMC abd.	70	67	63	60	56	53	49	46	42	39	35	32	28	25	21	18	14	11	7	4
MCP flex.	50	48	45	43	40	38	35	33	30	28	25	23	20	18	15	13	10	8	5	3
IP flex.	80	76	72	68	64	60	56	52	48	44	40	36	32	28	24	20	17	12	8	4
Digits 2–5																				
MCP flex.	90	86	81	77	72	68	63	59	54	50	45	41	36	32	27	23	18	14	9	5
MCP hypext.	45	43	41	38	36	34	32	29	27	25	23	20	18	16	14	11	9	7	5	2
MCP abd.	45	43	41	38	36	34	32	29	27	25	23	20	18	16	14	11	9	7	5	2
PIP flex.	100	95	90	85	80	75	70	65	60	55	50	45	40	35	30	25	20	15	10	5
DIP flex.	90	86	81	77	72	68	63	59	54	50	45	41	36	32	27	23	18	14	9	5
DIP hypext.	10	9	9	9	8	8	7	7	6	6	5	5	4	4	3	3	2	2	1	1

continues

Manual Muscle Testing—Hip and Knee				
Joint	Motion	Muscle(s)	Gravity+ Fair	Gravity− Poor
Hip	Flexion	Iliopsoas Rectus femoris Pectineus Tensor fas. latae Sartorius	Sitting	Sidelying
	Extension	Gluteus maximus Hamstrings	Prone Prone	Sidelying
	Abduction	Gluteus medius Gluteus minimus	Sidelying	Supine
	Adduction	Adductor longus Adductor brevis Adductor magnus	Sidelying	Supine

Manual Muscle Testing—Hip and Knee, cont.

Joint	Motion	Muscle(s)	Gravity+ Fair	Gravity— Poor
		Gracilis		
		Pectineus		
	Lateral Rot.	Piriformis	Sitting	Supine
		Gemellus sup./inf.		
		Obturator ext./int.		
		Quadratus fem.		
		Gluteus maximus		
	Medial Rot.	Gluteus minimus	Sitting	Supine
		Gluteus medius		
		Tensor fas. lat.		
Knee	Extension	Quadriceps	Sitting	Sidelying
	Flexion	Hamstrings	Prone	Sidelying
		Gastrocnemius		

Manual Muscle Testing—Ankle				
Joint	Motion	Muscle(s)	Gravity+ Fair	Gravity– Poor
Ankle	Dorsiflexion	Tibialis anterior Peroneus tertius Ext. digit long. Ext. hal. long.	Sitting	Sitting
	Plantar Flexion	Gastrocnemius Soleus	Standing	Prone
	Plantar Flexion	Soleus	Standing (with knee flexion)	Prone (with 90° knee flexion)
	Inversion	Tibialis posterior Tibialis anterior Flex. digit. long.	Sitting	Sitting

continues

Manual Muscle Testing—Ankle, cont.

Joint	Motion	Muscle(s)	Gravity+ Fair	Gravity— Poor
		Flex. hal. long. Ext. hal. long.		
	Eversion	Peroneus longus Peroneus brevis	Sitting	Sitting

Manual Muscle Testing—Shoulder

Joint	Motion	Muscle(s)	Gravity+ Fair	Gravity— Poor
Shoulder	Abduction	Deltoid Supraspinatus	Sitting	Supine
	Extension	Deltoid Latissimus dorsi Teres major	Prone	Sidelying

continues

Manual Muscle Testing—Shoulder, cont.

Joint	Motion	Muscle(s)	Gravity+ Fair	Gravity– Poor
	Flexion	Deltoid Coracobrachialis Pectoralis major	Sitting	Sidelying
	Horizon. Abd.	Deltoid Teres minor Infraspinatus	Prone	Sitting
	Horizon. Add.	Deltoid Pectoralis major	Supine	Sitting
	Lateral Rot.	Teres minor Infraspinatus Deltoid	Prone	Prone (with elbow ext.)

Manual Muscle Testing—Shoulder, cont.

Joint	Motion	Muscle(s)	Gravity+ Fair	Gravity– Poor
	Medial Rot.	Deltoid Latissimus dorsi Teres major Pectoralis major Subscapularis	Prone	Prone (with elbow ext.)

Manual Muscle Testing—Elbow and Wrist

Joint	Motion	Muscle(s)	Gravity+ Fair	Gravity– Poor
Elbow Complex	Flexion	Biceps Brachialis Brachioradialis	Sitting	Sitting (with 90° of shld. abd.)
	Extension	Triceps Anconeus	Prone (with 90° of shld. abd.)	Sitting (with 90° of shld. abd.)

Manual Muscle Testing—Elbow and Wrist, cont.

Joint	Motion	Muscle(s)	Gravity+ Fair	Gravity− Poor
	Supination	Biceps Supinator	Sitting (with 90° of elbow flex.)	Sitting (with 45°–90° of shld. flex. and 90° of elbow flex.)
	Pronation	Pronator teres Pronator quad.	Sitting (with 90° of elbow flex.)	Sitting (with 45°–90° of shld. flex. and 90° of elbow flex.)
Wrist	Extension	Ext. c. rad. long. Ext. c. rad. brev. Ext. c. ulnaris	Sitting (with forearm pronation and elbow flex.)	Sitting (with neutral forearm and elbow flex.)
	Flexion	Flex. carpi uln. Flex. carpi rad. Palmaris longus	Sitting (with forearm supination and elbow flex.)	Sitting (with neutral forearm and elbow flex.)

Special Tests Listing

Joint	Test Name	Assessment
Shoulder	Apprehension Test	anterior glenohumeral instability
	Clunk Sign	labral disorder
	Drop Arm Test	rotator cuff tear
	Hawkins-Kennedy Impingement Test	supraspinatus tendon impingement
	Impingement Sign	impingement of the supraspinatus and/or long head of biceps
	Lock Test	supraspinatus tendon impingement
	Neer Impingement Sign	subacromial impingement
	O'Brien Test	superior labral tear
	Speed's Maneuver	biceps tendon instability or tendonitis
	Yergason's Test	biceps tendon instability or tendonitis
Elbow	Cozen's Test	lateral epicondylitis
	Elbow Flexion Test	cubital tunnel syndrome
	Golfer's Elbow Test	medial epicondylitis
	Mill's Test	lateral epicondylitis
	Tinel's Sign at elbow	ulnar nerve entrapment

Special Tests Listing, cont.

Joint	Test Name	Assessment
Wrist and Hand	Allen Test	radial and ulnar artery circulation
	Bunnel-Littler Test	tightness of intrinsic muscles
	Carpal Shake Test	intercarpal synovitis
	Finkelstein's Test	stenosing tenosynovitis of abductor pollicis longus and extensor pollicis brevis
	Froment's Sign	ulnar nerve entrapment of elbow and wrist
	Murphy's Sign	lunate dislocation
	Phalen's Test	carpal tunnel syndrome
	Tinel's Test	carpal tunnel syndrome
Hip	90–90 Straight Leg Raise	hamstring tightness
	Craig Test	assess femoral anteversion or retroversion
	Ely's Test	flexibility of rectus femoris
	FABER or Patrick's Test	hip, lumbar, sacroiliac joint dysfunction or iliopsoas spasm
	Fulcrum Test	stress fracture of the femoral shaft
	Ober Test	tightness of iliotibial band and tensor fascia lata

continues

Special Tests Listing, cont.

Joint	Test Name	Assessment
Hip	Piriformis Test	tightness of the piriformis muscle
	Pelvic Drop Test	unstable hip of weak external rotators
	Quadrant (Scour) Test	capsular tightness, an adhesion, myofascial restriction or loss of joint congruity
	Thomas Test	decreased flexibility of rectus femoris or iliopsoas
	Trendelenburg Sign	weakness of gluteus medius
Knee	Anterior Draw Test	ACL and medial and posterior-medial capsuloligamentous instability
	Apley's Test	lesion of meniscus
	Apley's Distraction Test	medial or lateral collateral ligament injury
	Gravity (Godfrey) Sign	PCL injury
	Hughston's Posterolateral Drawer Test	posterolateral instability
	Lachman's Test	ACL injury
	McMurray's Test	lesion of medial meniscus
	Posterior Draw	PCL injury

continues

Special Tests Listing, cont.

Joint	Test Name	Assessment
Ankle	Buerger's Test	poor anterior circulation
	Fleiss Line	height of the medial arch
	Gungor Test	anterior displacement of the talus
	Homan's Sign	deep-vein thrombosis
	Kleiger Test	integrity of medial (deltoid) ligament
	Matles Test	chronic Achilles tendon rupture
	Morton's Test	presence of neuroma or a stress fracture
	Thompson Test	acute Achilles tendon rupture
Cranio-vertebral	Barre's Test	vertebral artery insufficiency
	Dix–Halpike Test	vestibular impairment–accumulation of utricle debris
	Modified Sharp-Purser Test	excessive translation of atlas
Cervical Spine	Compression Test	brachial plexus injury
	Hyperabduction Maneuver (Wright Test)	thoracic outlet compression

Special Tests Listing, cont.

Joint	Test Name	Assessment
Cervical Spine	Spurling's Test Stress Test	nerve root irritability brachial plexus injury
Sacroiliac Joint	Gaenslen's Test Yeoman's Test	sacroiliac lesion, hip pathology, or L4 nerve root lesion problem at the sacroiliac joint

Selected Special Tests Descriptions

Name	Assessment	Positive Test
SHOULDER **Drop Arm Test**	Positive test may indicate rotator cuff tear.	Abduct the shoulder against gravity. Instruct patient to slowly lower arm to side. The patient will not be able to lower arm smoothly and slowly; the arm will drop.

Selected Special Tests Descriptions, cont.

Name	Assessment	Positive Test
Hawkins-Kennedy Test	Positive test may indicate impingement syndrome involving the supraspinatus.	Flex the shoulder and elbow to 90° then internally rotate the shoulder. The patient will complain of pain.
Impingement Sign	Positive test may indicate impingement of the supraspinatus and/or long head of the biceps.	When sitting, passively horizontally adduct the shoulder with arm in 90° of shoulder flexion. Patient will have pain at the end range.
Neer Test	Positive test may indicate shoulder impingement involving the biceps tendon.	Passively and forcibly flex the shoulder. Patent will complain of pain.
Speed's Test	Positive test may indicate bicipital tendonitis.	Flex the shoulder against gravity about 60° with the elbow extended and forearm supinated.

continues

Selected Special Tests Descriptions, cont.

Name	Assessment	Positive Test
Yergason's Test	Postive test may indicate bicipital tendonitis.	Isometrically resist shoulder flexion at the forearm. Patient will complain of pain at the bicipital groove. Position the shoulder at the side and flex the elbow to 90° and pronate the forearm. Resist supination and external rotation. Patient will complain of pain at the bicipital groove.
Elbow		
Golfer's Elbow Test	Positive test may indicate medial epicondylitis.	Stabilize the elbow. Supinate the patient's forearm while extending the elbow and wrist. Patient will complain of pain at the medial epicondyle.
Mill's Test	Positive test may indicate lateral epicondylitis.	Stabilize the elbow. Ask the patient to pronate the forearm and extend and radially deviate the wrist against manual resistance. Patient will complain of pain at the lateral epicondyle.

continues

Selected Special Tests Descriptions, cont.

Name	Assessment	Positive Test
ELBOW		
Tinel's Test	Positive test may indicate a problem with the ulnar nerve.	Flex the elbow to 90°. Tap over the ulnar nerve.
		Patient will complain of paresthesias along the ulnar nerve sensory distribution.
WRIST		
Bunnel-Littler Test	Positive test may indicate tightness of the intrinsic muscles of the hand or a capsular problem of the joints.	Hold the MCP in extension and move the PIP into flexion. The PIP will not be able to be flexed.
Phalen's Test	Positive test may indicate carpal tunnel syndrome.	The patient flexes both wrists and presses the dorsal surfaces against each other to maintain flexion for 1 minute. The patient will experience paresthesias along the median nerve sensory distribution.

Selected Special Tests Descriptions, cont.

Name	Assessment	Positive Test
Tinel's Sign	Positive test may indicate lateral epicondylitis.	Supinate the forearm. Tap over the median nerve. The patient will experience paresthesias along the median nerve sensory distribution.
HIP		
Ober Test	Positive test may indicate tightness of the illiotibial band or tensor fascia latae.	Position the patient in sidelying on the uninvolved limb. Abduct and extend the uphill hip, then release the limb. The limb will not lower to the uninvolved limb.
Piriformis Test	Positive test may indicate tightness of the piriformis muscle.	Position the patient in sidelying on the uninvolved limb. Flex the hip to 60°–90° and the knee to 90°. Stabilize the pelvis and adduct the hip to the table. The patient will complain of pain in the buttocks.
Thomas Test	Positive test may indicate hip flexion contracture.	Place patient in supine. Have patient flex both hips and knees to the chest. Instruct patient to extend one limb to the table. The patient will be unable to fully extend the limb.

continues

Selected Special Tests Descriptions, cont.

Name	Assessment	Positive Test
Trendelenburg Sign	Positive test may indicate weakness of the gluteus medius.	Have patient stand on one leg. The pelvis will drop to the noninvolved side.
KNEE		
90–90 Straight Leg Raise Test	Positive test may indicate tightness of the hamstrings.	In supine, have the patient flex the hip and knee to 90°. Using the patient's or clinician's hands to maintain hip flexion, extend knee as much as possible. Patient is unable to extend knee beyond −20° extension.
ANKLE		
Apley's (Compression) Test	Positive test may indicate meniscus damage.	Have the patient assume the prone position and flex the knee to 90°. With the clinician's hands on the plantar surface of the foot, internally and externally rotate the leg while pressing down. Patient will complain of pain at the knee.

Selected Special Tests Descriptions, cont.

Name	Assessment	Positive Test
Apley's Distraction Test	Positive test may indicate collateral ligament damage.	Have the patient assume the prone position and flex the knee to 90°. Use one hand to grasp the leg just proximal to the malleoli and distract the leg while the other hand stabilizes at the posterior thigh. Patient will complain of pain at the knee.

Vital Signs

Note: Normal values may vary from one lab to another. The values presented in these charts should not be considered absolute.

Vital Sign	Age Group	Normal Range
Heart Rate (Pulse)	Newborns	70–190 beats/min
	1 yr	80–160 beats/min
	2–6 yrs	70–125 beats/min
	8–12 yrs	70–110 beats/min
	13–16 yrs	60–100 beats/min
	Adults	55–100 beats/min
Blood Pressure	Birth–1 mon	Systolic: 60–90 mm Hg
		Diastolic: 30–60 mm Hg
	2 mon–36 mon	Systolic: 75–130 mm Hg
		Diastolic: 45–90 mm Hg
	36 mon–adult	Systolic: 90–140 mm Hg
		Diastolic: 50–80 mm Hg

continues

Vital Signs, cont.

Note: Normal values may vary from one lab to another. The values presented in these charts should not be considered absolute.

Vital Sign	Age Group	Normal Range
Respiratory Rate	Birth to 1 mon	35–55 breaths/min
	3 mos. to 6 yrs	20–30 breaths/min
	6–10 yrs	15–25 breaths/min
	10–16 yrs	12–30 breaths/min
	Adults	12–20 breaths/min
Oxygen Saturation (as measured with a pulse oximiter)		Normal oxygen saturation at rest or during exercise is 98%. Exercise may be contra-indicated in values ≤90%.

References

American Spinal Injury Association. (2005). *International standard for neurological classification of spinal cord injury*. Chicago: ASIA.

Dutton, M. (2004). *Orthopedic examination, evaluation and intervention*. Philadelphia: McGraw Hill.

Goodman, C., Boissonault, W., & Fuller, K. (2003). *Pathology: Implications for the physical therapist*. Philadelphia: Saunders.

Hislop, H., & Montgomery, J. (2002). *Daniels and Worthingham's muscle testing: Techniques of manual examination*. Philadelphia: W.B. Saunders Company.

Hoppenfeld, S. (1976). *Physical examination of the spine and extremities.* Norwalk, CT: Prentice Hall.

Norkin, C., & White, J. (2003). *Measurement of joint motion: A guide to goniometry*. Philadelphia: F.A. Davis.

Palmer, L., & Epler, M. (1998). *Fundamentals of musculoskeletal assessment techniques.* Philadelphia: Lippincott.

2

Therapeutic Modalities

Cryotherapy

Description
Cryotherapy is the use of cold to achieve therapeutic results.

Indications
Cryotherapy is typically used for pain management, anti-inflammation, edema control, decrease of muscle guarding/spasm, spasticity management.

Administration Techniques
Ice massage: Ice massage can easily and quickly anesthetize a local region of the skin. It is typically applied using an "ice pop" or water frozen in a paper cup. The ice is applied directly to the skin over the target area.

Cold packs: Cold packs are typically applied to relatively large surface areas and around joints. They are helpful in reducing inflammation and pain. Cold packs are not applied directly to the skin. A moist towel between the cold pack and skin maximizes heat transfer.

Cooling + Compression Devices: There are several devices on the market that combine compression and cooling by circulating chilled water through a compression cuff wrapped around a joint or limb segment. Edema control is

continues

Cryotherapy, cont.

Administration Techniques	provided via the compression. The closed insulated environment containing the chilled water minimizes warming and therefore provides a more consistent and prolonged cooling.
Treatment Considerations	Patient sensation tolerance to cryotherapy is quite variable. The clinician must be very attentive to patient reports.
	Typical sensation progression during cryotherapy includes cold → stinging → aching → anesthesia. Often patients do not tolerate the aching stage.
	It is important to specifically target the desired tissue to ensure effectiveness. Treatment time is typically 10–15 minutes.
Critical Assessment Parameters	Pretreatment assessment of skin condition and careful assessment of skin reaction should be undertaken.
	Normal response to cryotherapy includes mild to moderate skin erythema.
	Signs and symptoms of too much cooling include severe pain, skin discoloration, itching and burning, blistering, and edema.
Effective Documentation Practices	Effective documentation includes careful description of the cryotherapy technique used, treatment location, length of treatment, and patient tolerance and reaction. If being used to manage pain, pre- and posttreatment pain scales should be documented.
Precautions and Contraindications	Cryotherapy should be cautiously used on patients with sensory deficits, circulatory impairment, cold hypersensitivity, and hypertension.

Fluidotherapy

Description	Fluidotherapy is a superficial heating modality that transfers heat by convection. Dried corn husks or other cellulose material are suspended by warmed circulating air. The specific heat of the suspended material and the air allow for higher therapeutic temperatures to be achieved.
Indications	Fluidotherapy is practically used when moderate to vigorous heating of the wrist and hand is indicated. It can also be used for the ankle and foot. Clinical indications include arthritis, chronic tendonitis, postoperative conditions, postfracture management, and Raynaud's syndrome.
Administration Techniques	The fluidotherapy machine must be preheated to the desired temperature. When at room temperature, it could take up to 40 minutes for the machine to reach the desired therapeutic temperature.
	The distal limb is placed inside of the fluidotherapy cabinet.
	Turbulence of the suspended particles can be controlled. Treatment time is typically 15–20 minutes.
Treatment Considerations	Clinician must account for potentially long preheating period. This heating modality allows for simultaneous heating and range of motion activities.
	The patient can manipulate nonmetal therapeutic devices such as rubber balls while receiving treatment. Additional entry ports allow the clinician to enter the cabinet and provide passive range of motion.

continues

Fluidotherapy, cont.

Critical Assessment Parameters	Pretreatment assessment of skin condition and careful assessment of skin reaction should be undertaken.
	Objective assessment of pain (pain scales) and range of motion is critical in gauging effectiveness.
	Posttreatment skin condition and patient response should be noted.
Effective Documentation Practices	Treatment time, temperature, and treatment area should be carefully documented. Objective documentation of the patient's report of pain, goniometric assessment, and skin condition is important.
	Subjective response related to "stiffness," other symptoms, and the patient's response to treatment should be documented.
Precautions and Contraindications	Fluidotherapy should be cautiously used in the presence of open wounds. Open wounds must be covered with a plastic barrier to prevent cellulose particles from entering the wound.

Iontophoresis

Description	In iontophoresis, a continuous direct current is used to transmit ions through the skin.
Indications	Iontophoresis is typically used for pain management, anti-inflammation, scar lysis, enhanced healing.
Administration Techniques	For safety purposes, iontophoresis is best provided using a device specifically designed for ion transfer. Many of these devices automatically adjust treatment time as current intensity changes.

Iontophoresis, cont.

Administration Techniques

Current intensity is typically measured in milliamps. Iontophoresis uses two electrodes: one active and one dispersive.

The clinician determines the polarity of the active electrode based upon the charge of the ions to be transferred.

Negative ions are transferred under the negative electrode and positive ions under the positive electrode. Dosage is expressed in milliamp-minutes (mA-min). For example, a dosage of 20 mA-min may be provided with an intensity of 4 mA applied for 5 minutes. The same dosage may be achieved with an intensity of 2 mA for 10 minutes. Typical dosages range from 20 to 40 mA-min with dosages dependent on the ion being transferred. Many treatment protocols exist.

Treatment Considerations

Iontophoresis is best applied to a specific, localized, and relatively superficial target tissue. Such tissues include rotator cuff tendons, common wrist/finger/hand flexor and extensor origins, patella ligament, Achilles tendon, etc.

Given the somewhat caustic nature of continuous direct current, the clinician should gradually increase intensity and remain within the patient's tolerance. The patient should only experience a mild tingling sensation.

The goal of the treatment should be kept in mind and appropriate assessment parameters established. The patient should be instructed to report any delayed posttreatment skin irritation immediately.

continues

Iontophoresis, cont.

Critical Assessment Parameters	Depending on the pathology, goals, and ion being transferred, if effective, positive results should be noted in one to three treatment sessions. Objective assessment of pain includes the use of questionnaires and visual analog scales.
Effective Documentation Practices	Careful notation of dosage, current intensity, ionic substance, and active electrode polarity is crucial.
	Specific descriptions of electrode placement are also necessary.
	Documentation should also include a description of pre- and posttreatment skin condition, patient's sensory tolerance, and posttreatment efficacy (using the most objective measures possible).
Precautions and Contraindications	Iontophoresis is contraindicated in areas with bruises, cuts, or otherwise broken skin. It is also contraindicated in acute injuries and over sites of active hemorrhage.
	General contraindications for electrical stimulation apply.
	Iontophoresis should be very cautiously applied in areas of impaired sensation.

Low-Level Laser Therapy

Description	Low-level laser therapy uses light energy to facilitate therapeutic effects at the cellular level. Though used extensively in Europe, it is an emerging modality in the United States. Lasers in the United States use helium neon (HeNe) gas or gallium arsenide (GaAs) as lasing mediums.

Low-Level Laser Therapy, cont.

Indications	The Food and Drug Administration has specifically approved the sale of laser devices for the treatment of pain in carpal tunnel syndrome. Laser therapy has been found to be effective in wound healing, the treatment of tendon and ligament injuries, edema control, and scar tissue inhibition.
Administration Techniques	**Gridding technique:** The treatment area is divided into a grid of square centimeters. The tip of the applicator is placed in light contact with the skin. Each grid is stimulated for a specified period of time. A sterile plastic grid sheet may be placed over open wounds to allow for applicator contact.
	Scanning technique: This technique is the same as gridding except the applicator does not make contact with the treatment site.
Treatment Considerations	Treatment protocols are not well defined. More research is required to determine optimal and standardized dosages.
Critical Assessment Parameters	Assessment is dictated by the goals of the treatment. Careful documentation of pain using pain scales is critical. Pre- and postcircumferential measurements assess edema control effectiveness.
Effective Documentation Practices	Dosage must be carefully documented. Lasing technique must also be clearly indicated.
Precautions and Contraindications	There are apparently very few adverse effects of low-level laser.
	When applied to the head or neck, the patient should wear protective goggles. For safety purposes, the clinician should wear protective goggles.

continues

Low-Level Laser Therapy, cont.

The modality should not be applied during the first trimester of pregnancy or over cancerous cells.

Mechanical Intermittent Compression

Description	Intermittent compression techniques use gravity and compressed air to facilitate lymphatic and general venous flow in the treatment of joint swelling and lymphedema.
Indications	Intermittent compression can be used to treat lymphedema, traumatic and chronic edema, and stasis ulcers.
Administration Techniques	Intermittent compression uses various inflatable extremity sleeves that are alternately filled and emptied of air exerting external pressure on an extremity.

There are several parameters under clinician control. They include:

Inflation pressure: Inflation pressures are administered between 30 mmHg and 80 mmHg dependent upon treatment goals and target extremity. Pressure dosage is closely correlated with blood pressure and patient comfort.

On/off cycle: On/off cycles may be variable and are protocol specific. On/off cycle refers to the amount of time the pressure is exerted versus the amount of time it is relieved.

Treatment time: Typical treatment time is 30 to 40 minutes.

Treatment Considerations	The limb should be elevated during treatment. The patient should have intact sensation and a reliable mental status.

Mechanical Intermittent Compression, cont.

Blood pressure should be taken prior to treatment. Pressures should not exceed systolic pressure.

Critical Assessment Parameters
Volumetric or limb girth measures effectively assess edema reductions.

Effective Documentation Practices
Circumferential measurements must be carefully documented. Measurement areas should be identified by referring to distances from bony landmarks.

Documentation of edema as a percentage comparison to the uninvolved extremity is effective.

Specific documentation of dosage, on/off cycle, and treatment time is required.

Precautions and Contraindications
Contraindications include deep-vein thrombosis, local infection, congestive heart failure, acute pulmonary edema, and displaced fractures.

Neuromuscular Electrical Stimulation (NMES)

Description
NMES uses electrical stimulation to activate muscle by stimulating an intact or partially intact peripheral nerve.

Functional electrical stimulation (FES) is a form of NMES. It is used as a substitute for an orthosis to stimulate paralyzed or paretic muscle.

NMES can be accomplished with a variety of electrical stimulators including low-voltage alternating current and high-voltage galvanic current stimulators.

Indications
NMES is typically used to treat muscle atrophy, muscle weakness, peripheral neuropathy, muscle spasm.

continues

Neuromuscular Electrical Stimulation (NMES), cont.

Administration Techniques

Bipolar technique: This technique concentrates current in the target area. It tends to facilitate an effective contraction of the target muscle group. It is appropriate when targeting muscle groups such as the quadriceps, wrist flexors/extensors, ankle dorsiflexors, etc. One active electrode and an equal-sized dispersive electrode are placed over the target musculature.

Monopolar technique: This technique concentrates current in a small, local target area. It is more appropriate when targeting a specific muscle rather than a group of muscles. This technique uses a single, small active or stimulating electrode placed over the target muscle. A second larger dispersive electrode is placed on the same side of the body away from the target area.

Treatment Considerations

Pulse amplitude/intensity: The strength or intensity of the current is one treatment parameter that influences the quality of the facilitated muscle contraction. Pulse amplitude is gradually increased within the patient's sensory tolerance limits. As physiological accommodation occurs, the patient usually can tolerate increased intensity. Sometimes it may take one to two sessions for patients to tolerate their maximal intensity.

Measured in Amperes (A)—low voltage and Milliamperes (mA)—low/high voltage.

Pulse rate/frequency: Generally, smooth, tetanic contractions are achieved with pulse rates greater than 35–50 pulses per second. Pulse rates

Neuromuscular Electrical Stimulation (NMES), cont.

will differ dependent on the goal of the treatment. Because higher frequencies influence sensory perception and levels of muscle fatigue, clinicians should select the lowest frequency that achieves the desired results.

Measured in pulses per second (pps) and Hertz (Hz).

Pulse duration/width: An inverse relationship exists between pulse duration and amplitude. Therefore, less amplitude is required with longer pulse widths. This relationship is helpful in achieving desired results within the patient's sensory limits.

Measured in milliseconds (mSec.).

Duty cycle: Duty cycle refers to the stimulation on/off ratio. This parameter is important in preventing muscle fatigue. Typically, clinical duty cycles are 1:3 (such as 5 seconds on and 15 seconds off) or 1:5 (such as 10 seconds on and 50 seconds off). On times rarely exceed 10 seconds.

Ramp: Ramp refers to the rate of rise to maximum pulse intensity or pulse width. Ramp may also include the rate of declination of intensity or width. In other words, the ramp function provides for a gradual change in pulse intensity or width rather than an instantaneous change. This parameter affects the quality of muscle contraction and sensory perception.

Measured in milliseconds (mSec.).

Critical Assessment Parameters
It is difficult to practically and objectively assess an electrically induced muscle contraction. Special emphasis should be placed on describing the quality of the muscle contraction, including

continues

Neuromuscular Electrical Stimulation (NMES), cont.

smoothness and specificity of joint motion achieved.

Effective Documentation Practices

Effective documentation includes a careful description of all parameters (intensity, width, etc.). Total treatment time should be noted. The use of tape measures and surface anatomy sites should be used in order to accurately document electrode placement.

Precautions and Contraindications

Electrical stimulation is generally contraindicated in pregnancy.

It is also contraindicated in the presence of a cardiac pacemaker or other implanted electrical stimulators.

Due to the risk of metastasis, electrical stimulation is contraindicated in the presence of cancer.

Other contraindications include in the presence of active tuberculosis, in an area of thrombophlebitis or thrombosis, over the carotid sinus, or in areas of active hemorrhage.

Precautions include obesity, impaired sensation, and over relatively superficial metal implants.

Paraffin Bath

Description

Paraffin baths provide superficial heat by coating the target area with solution of melted paraffin wax and mineral oil.

Indications

Paraffin is typically used for the treatment of chronic arthritis of the hand and foot. It may also be used in the treatment of various distal extremity conditions to increase ROM and to manage pain.

Paraffin Bath, cont.

Administration Techniques	The most popular and safer technique for the administration of paraffin treatment is called the dip technique. In this technique, the distal extremity is coated with 8 to 12 coats of paraffin.
	The distal extremity is then wrapped in plastic and then a terry towel. The patient is positioned so that the extremity is elevated. The paraffin glove remains in place for 15 to 20 minutes.
Treatment Considerations	Paraffin provides heat at temperatures between 126°F and 128°F. This high temperature increases the risk of burn. The lower specific heat of paraffin allows for the higher therapeutic temperatures.
	Some patients are unable to tolerate the high therapeutic temperatures.
	Paraffin does not allow for inspection of the skin during the treatment.
Critical Assessment Parameters	Objective assessment of pain (pain scales), skin condition/response, and range of motion is critical in gauging effectiveness.
Effective Documentation Practices	Documentation must include pre-post skin treatment condition, objective pain and range of motion parameters, and patient's subjective reports.
	Careful documentation of circumferential measurements, including descriptions of distances from bony landmarks is important.
Precautions and Contraindications	All general precautions and contraindications to heat apply to paraffin. Paraffin is clearly contraindicated in the presence of open wounds.

continues

Transcutaneous Electrical Nerve Stimulation (TENS)

Description	Typically, TENS is used to stimulate sensory and/or motor nerves in an effort to manage pain. It is thought that this modality is effective through the application of the gate control theory of pain, the stimulation of the release of endogenous opiates, and/or the central biasing theory. Although TENS is associated with specific compact portable units, its pain relief effects can be achieved using a variety of electrical stimulators.
Indications	Indications include chronic pain syndrome, spinal radiculopathy, low back pain, reflex sympathetic dystrophy, etc.
Administration Techniques	**Gate Control**: This technique uses high pulse rate, low pulse width.
	Endogenous Opiates: This technique uses high intensity, low pulse width, low pulse rate.
	Central Biasing: This technique uses very high intensity, high pulse width, high pulse rate.
Treatment Considerations	TENS is principally designed as an ambulatory modality. Patients should be allowed to ambulate, perform ADL, and occupational tasks while the modality is administered.
	If one of these techniques is not effective, clinician should systematically trial an alternative technique.
	Effectiveness may also be dependent on electrode placement that may include several configurations.

Transcutaneous Electrical Nerve Stimulation (TENS), cont.

If effective, pain modulation is apparent within 2–30 minutes of administration. Sensory accommodation may decrease effectiveness.

In an effort to minimize physiological accommodation, many TENS units have an optional modulation mode that alternately changes treatment parameters thereby decreasing accommodation potential.

Critical Assessment Parameters	Careful attempts to objectively assess pain are critical in determining effectiveness. The use of pain ratings, visual analogs, and questionnaires provide the basis for pre- and posttreatment assessments.
Effective Documentation Practices	Effective documentation practices include specific notation of technique, frequency, pulse width, intensity changes, electrode placement, and treatment time. Pre- and posttreatment pain assessments should be carefully noted.
Precautions and Contraindications	TENS may interfere with demand type pacemakers and therefore is contraindicated when present.
	It should not be administered over the carotid sinus, a pregnant uterus, and the head and neck of epileptics.

Ultrasound

Description	Ultrasound is a deep heating modality. Sound waves at extremely low intensity and very high frequency are introduced to tissue producing thermal and nonthermal effects.
Indications	Ultrasound is used to increase the extensibility of collagen fibers in tendons and joint capsules, reduce muscle spasm, and modulate pain.

continues

Ultrasound, cont.

Nonthermal effects may positively affect healing in damaged tissue, by altering the permeability of cells.

Administration Techniques

Several ultrasound treatment parameters are under clinician control. They include intensity, frequency, treatment time, and waveform.

Typical intensity: .75 to 1.5 W/cm^2

Frequency: 1MHz for deep penetration or 3MHz for less deep penetration

Treatment time: 5 to 10 minutes

Waveform: Continuous wave for thermal and nonthermal effects or pulsed for primarily nonthermal effects

Treatment Considerations

Liberal use of conducting gel is required.

Underwater technique should be used when treating uneven surfaces.

Specific and limited treatment area should be identified. Larger areas require longer treatment times.

The sound head must remain in full contact with the gel at a 90° angle to the skin.

When applying ultrasound to increase range of motion, position the patient for simultaneous stretching, if possible.

The patient should not perceive heat. If the sound head becomes excessively warm, the clinician should add additional gel and maintain good skin contact. If the problem persists, the unit should be checked by a biomedical technician.

Ultrasound, cont.

	Sign of overdosage is the patient's complaint of sudden and sharp pain in the treatment area. Some patients complain of a gradually increasing ache.
Critical Assessment Parameters	Objective assessment of pain (pain scales) and range of motion is critical in gauging effectiveness.
Effective Documentation Practices	Documentation of specific target tissue, intensity, treatment time, and waveform are critical for enhancing reproducibility.
Precautions and Contraindications	Ultrasound is contraindicated in areas of decreased circulation or impaired sensation and over the reproductive organs or eyes. It is also contraindicated over a pregnant uterus, pacemaker, or in the presence of malignancy. Ultrasound may be contraindicated over total joint replacements and active epiphyseal growth plates.

References

Behrens, B., & Michlovitz, S. (2006). *Physical agents: Theory and practice*. Philadelphia: F.A. Davis.

Hecox, B., Mehreteab, T., Weisberg, J., & Sanko, J. (2006). *Integrating physical agents in rehabilitation*. Upper Saddle River, NJ: Pearson Prentice Hall.

Prentice, W.E. (2005). *Therapeutic modalities in rehabilitation*. New York: McGraw Hill.

Therapeutic Exercise

Closed Kinetic Chain Exercises	
Joint	Exercise Description
Shoulder	**Patient Position:** Standing

Activity: The patient leans against the wall with elbows extended. The clinician applies alternating, multidirectional resistance to the trunk and pelvis while the patient is instructed to attempt to hold his or her position.

Progression: In the same position, place a medium-sized therapeutic ball between the patient and the wall, then apply the same alternating multidirectional resistance to the trunk and pelvis.

Patient Position: Quadruped

Activity: Place a rocker or balance board in front of the patient. The patient places both hands on the rocker or balance board with extended elbows. The patient then performs weight-shifting activities.

Patient Position: Quadruped with therapeutic ball supporting the trunk

Activity: Weight bearing on hands and through extended elbows, patient performs weight-shifting activities.

continues

Closed Kinetic Chain Exercises, cont.

Joint	Exercise Description
Elbow	**Patient Position**: Standing
	Activity: Patient performs push-ups while leaning against the wall.
	Progression: In sitting, patient performs push-ups while holding onto chair arms or parallel bars.
Hip	**Patient Position**: Supine
	Activity: Patient flexes both hips and knees so that the plantar surfaces of both feet are in contact with the supporting surface. Patient then pushes the feet into supporting surface and lifts the buttocks.
	Progression: The patient performs same activity with one LE or with manual resistance applied at the pelvis.
Knee	**Patient Position**: Standing
	Activity: Loop elastic resistive around the patient's pelvis. The patient ambulates against the resistance of the elastic with emphasis on knee flexion.
	Patient Position: Standing
	Activity: The patient stands with one limb ahead of the other. Keeping both feet in position, the patient lunges forward by flexing the trunk and allowing the front knee flexion.
	Progression: Increase distance between the extremities, allow knee flexion to approach 90°.
	Patient Position: Standing
	Activity: The patient stands with the back against a wall. While maintaining trunk extension, the patient flexes the hips and knees to slide down the wall and then extends the joints to slide back up the wall.

Closed Kinetic Chain Exercises, cont.

Joint	Exercise Description

Progression: Place a therapeutic ball between the wall and patient's back and perform the activity.

Patient Position: Standing

Activity: The patient performs partial squats allowing knee flexion to 30° to 40°.

Progression: Increase the amount of knee flexion.

Patient Position: Standing

Activity: Loop elastic resistive around an immovable object. Place one end of the loop around the proximal posterior leg. Position the patient so the elastic resistive is near maximal stretch. The patient then performs the slow-count squat activity.

Patient Position: Standing

Activity: The patient faces a 2- to 3-inch step. Patient places one foot on the step and brings the other foot up. In the same position, the patient first flexes the knee and extends the hip, then brings the foot back to the floor.

Progression: Increase the height of the step.

Patient Position: Sitting on rolling chair or stool or in a wheelchair

Activity: With the feet remaining on the supporting surface and knees initially at 90° of flexion, use the lower extremities to push or pull a chair through a therapeutic cone obstacle course.

Progression: Alter the obstacle course. Add friction brakes to the wheels or perform the activity in stocking feet to reduce friction.

continues

Closed Kinetic Chain Exercises, cont.

Joint	Exercise Description
Ankle	**Patient Position**: Sitting
	Activity: The patient places one or both feet on a rocker or balance board. Maintaining knee extension of the weight-bearing limb(s), the patient weight shifts in a manner to cause a variety of ankle motions.
	Progression: Perform the same activity in supported standing.

Frenkel's Exercise

Frenkel's exercises are a series of motions of increasing difficulty performed by ataxic patients to facilitate the restoration of coordination.

Position	Movement Activity Instructions
Supine	Lying on bed, bend your right leg to your chest. Return your right leg to the start position and repeat this activity with your left leg. Perform this activity 10 times.
	Bend your knees so that your feet are flat on the bed. Spread your right leg apart and then back to the center and repeat this activity with your left leg. Perform this activity 10 times.
	Lift your right leg and left arm together and then return to the start position. Lift your left leg and right arm and then return to start position. Perform this activity 10 times.
	Place your right heel on your left kneecap and then return it to the start position. Place your left heel on your right kneecap and return to starting position. Perform this activity 10 times.
	Slide your right heel along your left leg up to the kneecap and then return to the start position. Slide

Frenkel's Exercise, cont.

Position	Movement Activity Instructions
	your left heel along your right leg up to the kneecap and then return to the start position. Perform this activity 10 times.
Sitting	Spread the objects out on the floor in front of you. Try to touch each object with your right foot and then with your left foot. Repeat this activity 10 times.
	Spread the objects out on a table in front of you. Try to touch each object with your right hand and then with your left hand. Repeat this activity 10 times.
	Stretch your right hand out from your body and then bring your index finger to your nose, then perform the same activity with your left hand. Repeat this activity 10 times.
	Pat the palms of your hands on your thighs and then pat the back of your hands on your thighs. Repeat this activity 10 times.
Quadruped	While on your hands and knees, lift your right leg and return it to start position. Lift your left leg and return it to the start position. Repeat this activity 10 times.
	While on your hands and knees, lift your right arm and return it to start position. Lift your left arm and return it to the start position. Repeat this activity 10 times.
	While on your hands and knees, lift your right leg and left arm, then return them to the start position. Lift your left leg and right arm, then return them to the start position. Repeat this activity 10 times.

continues

Frenkel's Exercise, cont.

Position	Movement Activity Instructions
Kneeling	While kneeling on both knees, alternately shift your weight from right to left. Repeat this activity 10 times.
	While kneeling on both knees, alternately walk forward and then backward. Repeat this activity 10 times.
	While kneeling on both knees, alternately lift your right and then your left leg so that the sole of each foot is placed on the floor. Repeat this activity 10 times.
Standing	Side step to the left for 10 steps, then side step to the right for 10 steps.
	Walk 10 steps forward by placing your right heel just in front of your left big toe and then your left heel in front of your right big toe.
	Walk 10 steps backwards by placing your right big toe just behind of your left heel and then your left big toe just behind your right heel.

Low Back Pain Exercises

Pain Syndrome	Exercise Interventions
Derangement Syndrome: This syndrome occurs as a result of an alteration to the normal resting position of two adjacent vertebrae secondary to a change in the position of the interspersed nucleus pulposis. Changes in pulposis position may lead to a varying degree of spinal cord, nerve root, or vascular compression.	**Extension Principle Activities** The general goal of these activities is to restore the nucleus pulposis to a more normal position. Typically, this goal may be subdivided into four phases: (1) reduction of the derangement, (2) maintenance of the reduction, (3) recovery of function, and (4) prevention of recurrence of symptoms. Lumbar extension activities are used to affect the fluid dynamics of the pulposis and move it to a more normal position.

Low Back Pain Exercises, cont.

Pain Syndrome	Exercise Interventions
	The patient lies in prone with arms at the trunk and head turned to either side. This position will facilitate some lumbar lordosis (extension). The patient maintains this position for about 5 minutes and then assumes a prone on the elbows position.
	In the prone on elbows position, the patient places the elbows under the shoulders and supports the upper half of the body while the pelvis and thighs remain on the supporting surface. It is important that the patient relaxes in this position, allowing the low back to sag. Lumbar muscular contraction will cause joint compression which may limit pulposis movement.
	Following this position, the patient should assume the prone position for 5–10 minutes and then progress to extension in lying.
	In the extension in lying position, the patient places the hands near the shoulder as if about to perform a traditional push-up. The patient then pushes the top half of the body up by extending the elbows while the pelvis and thighs remain on the supporting surface. This activity is performed in three to four sets of 10.
	These activities may be performed in a progression or individually, dependent on the behavior and extent of the symptoms.

continues

Low Back Pain Exercises, cont.

Pain Syndrome	Exercise Interventions
	The goal of the activities is to centralize or reduce radiating symptoms and ultimately reduce local back pain.
	A wide belt may be used to stabilize the pelvis during extension in lying exercises.
Flexion Dysfunction Syndrome: Dysfunction syndrome occurs as a result of maladaptive shortening of spinal soft tissue precipitating a loss of mobility. Soft tissues are prematurely elongated before full range of motion is achieved. The premature stretching of these tissues causes pain. Flexion dysfunction is common and involves loss of lumbar flexion range of motion.	Treatment of dysfunction requires the elongation or stretching of shortened soft tissue. Therefore, it is important to educate the patient that initial treatment may actually seem to worsen or at least aggravate symptoms because it is premature elongation of these structures that cause pain. Flexion dysfunction is treated with the flexion principle. Flexion activities stretch shortened posterior spinal soft tissues that limit flexion. In flexion in lying, the patient lies supine with the knees and hips flexed so that the feet are flat on the supporting surface. The patient then flexes the hips and knees toward the chest and uses the hands to pull the anterior thighs close to the chest. This position is held for 10–15 seconds and then the patient returns to the starting position. This exercise is repeated 10 times. In flexion in standing, the patient maintains knee extension and flexes at the hip reaching toward the toes. This position is held for 5–10 seconds and

Low Back Pain Exercises, cont.

Pain Syndrome	Exercise Interventions
	then the patient returns to upright standing. This activity is repeated 10 times.
	In flexion step standing, the patient stands on one leg while the other foot is placed on the seat of a stool or chair with the hip and knee flexed to about 90°. Maintaining extension of the weight-bearing limb, the patient flexes the trunk progressing toward the shoulder being lower than the flexed knee. The patient holds this position for 10–15 seconds and then returns to the start position. This activity is repeated 6 to 10 times.
Extension Dysfunction Syndrome: Dysfunction syndrome occurs as a result of maladaptive shortening of spinal soft tissue precipitating a loss of mobility. Soft tissues are prematurely elongated before full range of motion is achieved. The premature stretching of these tissues causes pain. Extension dysfunction is the most common form of dysfunction and involves the loss of lumbar extension range of motion.	Treatment of dysfunction requires the elongation or stretching of shortened soft tissue. Therefore, it is important to educate the patient that initial treatment may actually seem to worsen or at least aggravate symptoms because it is premature elongation of these structures that cause pain. Extension dysfunction is treated with the extension principle. Passive extension activities stretch shortened anterior spinal soft tissues that limit extension. Passive extension activities used in derangement syndrome are used in the treatment of extension dysfunction.

continues

Low Back Pain Exercises, cont.

Pain Syndrome	Exercise Interventions

Postural Syndrome (sitting): This syndrome occurs when the lumbar spine is held in a relatively static position. Soft tissues surrounding the bony structures are placed under prolonged stress. In postural syndrome, the patient only complains of symptoms when the stressful posture is assumed.

Slouch–Overcorrect

The goal of this activity is to sensitize the patient to the extremes of poor and optimal sitting posture.

Description: While sitting on a backless stool, the patient assumes an exaggerated slouched position—reversed lumbar lordosis and forward head posture. After maintaining this position for 10–15 seconds, the patient assumes an exaggerated corrected position—lumbar lordosis, shoulders posterior, and exaggerated cervical lordosis.

These two postures are then alternately assumed in a rhythmical pattern. After performing this activity, the patient is able to easily assume the extreme optimum posture.

The patient is instructed to assume the extreme optimum position whenever they feel pain.

The patient is then taught to assume this position and then to partially relax so that an optimum but not extreme posture is assumed.

Postural Syndrome (standing)

Slouch–Overcorrect

The goal of this exercise is to sensitize the patient to the extreme of poor posture in order to enhance postural correction.

Low Back Pain Exercises, cont.

Pain Syndrome	Exercise Interventions
	Description: There are two major standing postures that may lead to low back pain. The patient is taught to assume and then correct one of these postures dependent on which one precipitates symptoms.
	Position 1: This standing position is assumed by instructing the patient to fold their arms across the abdomen and allowing the chest to drop. The thoracic spine moves posteriorly and the pelvis moves anteriorly placing the lumbar-sacral joints in full extension.
	Position 2: This standing position is assumed by instructing the patient by weight shifting all body weight onto one limb, while the knee of the other limb is allowed to flex. This causes the pelvis to move anteriorly and the lumbar-sacral joints into extension.
	The patient becomes sensitized to the extremes of the corrected and poor postures and learns how to assume more normal relatively pain-free postures.

Postamputation Exercises

Transfemoral Amputation/AKA	• Quad sets • Hip flexion in supine, sitting and standing (manual/weight resistance) • Hip extension in sidelying and prone (manual resistance) • Unilateral bridging • Hip abduction Progressing Exercises: • Use elastic resistives to resist motions • Add weights or manual resistance at pelvis during bridges
Transtibial Amputation/BKA	• All exercises for transfemoral amputees • Straight-leg raises • Hip extension (prone) with knee flexion • Hip extension (prone) with knee extension • Knee flexion (manual resistance) in prone/sitting

• All standing exercises should be performed in the parallel bars or with UE support and supervision.

• Emphasis must be placed on the maintenance and improvement of the range of motion and strength of both extremities.

• Range-of-motion considerations are especially critical for ADL and prosthetic fit.

• Upper extremity strength should be generally addressed.

• Therapeutic activities should emphasize weight shifting to the involved side with appropriate stabilizing contractions.

Proprioceptive Neuromuscular Facilitation (PNF)

Description	PNF is a therapeutic exercise technique that promotes or hastens neuromuscular responses by stimulating proprioceptors. The technique uses diagonal movement patterns rather than more traditional cardinal plane motions.
Supporting Theory	The theory that supports the use of PNF states that each segment of the body moves in specific diagonals that allow for maximal contraction. These diagonals are considered the basis for all normal movement.
	The theory suggests that PNF is a more effective exercise technique by positing the notion that the cerebral cortex does not deal with isolated motor activity, but only with mass movement patterns from which isolated movement is derived. By exercising in diagonal patterns, muscles are strengthened or facilitated in a more functional manner.
PNF Benefits	Increased strength of contraction
	Facilitation of normal motion in patients with neurological deficits
	Increased coordination
	Increased endurance
	Increased ROM
Treatment Consideration	The clinician must provide accurate and comfortable sensory stimulation during exercise; hand placement is important.
	Proper hand placement and manual contact allow for appropriate provision of resistance, facilitation of specific muscle groups, and movement guidance.

continues

Proprioceptive Neuromuscular Facilitation (PNF), cont.

	Manual resistance can be applied to selective components of diagonal movement patterns dependent on the patient's needs.
	Verbal instructions must be clear, concise, and in lay terms.
	For PNF to be most effective, the patient must have normal vision and hearing, good cognitive skills, and intact sensory mechanisms.
	Primary (D1) and secondary (D2) patterns can be used in a treatment progression. Secondary patterns require greater voluntary control. They can be used to develop increased selectivity and coordination.
Disadvantages	The use of manual resistance hampers the ability to provide objective measures of progress. However, even if PNF is being used, the clinician can still rely on manual muscle testing and dynamometry to assess strength of individual muscle groups.
	PNF may be more time consuming because it requires clinician contact during the entire exercise session.

PNF Diagonal Patterns

Pattern	Start Position	End Position	Commands
UE Diagonal 1 (D1) Flexion (with elbow extension)	• Fingers and wrist extended • Forearm pronation • Elbow extension • Shoulder extension abduction int. rot.	• Fingers and wrist flexed • Forearm supination • Elbow extended • Shoulder flexion adduction ext. rot.	Squeeze my hand, turn your palm up, and pull my hand across your face keeping your elbow straight.
UE Diagonal 1 (D1) Extension (with elbow extension)	• Fingers and wrist flexion • Forearm supination • Elbow extension • Shoulder flexion adduction ext. rot.	• Fingers and wrist extension • Forearm pronation • Elbow extension • Shoulder extension abduction int. rot.	Open your hand, turn your palm down, push down and away from your face keeping your elbow straight.
UE Diagonal 2 (D2) Flexion (with elbow extension)	• Fingers and wrist flexion • Forearm pronation • Elbow extension • Shoulder extension adduction int. rot.	• Fingers and wrist extension • Forearm supination • Elbow extension • Shoulder flexion abduction ext. rot.	Open your hand, turn your palm up, and lift up and out toward me keeping your elbow straight.

continues

PNF Diagonal Patterns, cont.

Pattern	Start Position	End Position	Commands
UE Diagonal 2 (D2) Extension (with elbow extension)	• Fingers and wrist extended • Forearm supination • Elbow extension • Shoulder flexion abduction ext. rot.	• Fingers and wrist flexion • Forearm pronation • Elbow extension • Shoulder flexion adduction int. rot.	Squeeze my hand, turn your palm down, pull down toward your opposite hip, keeping your elbow straight.
LE Diagonal 1 (D1) Flexion (with knee extension)	• Plantar flexion • Eversion • Knee ext. • Hip extension abduction int. rot.	• Dorsiflexion • Inversion • Knee ext. • Hip flexion adduction ext. rot.	Turn your heel in and pull your foot up and across your body keeping your knee straight.
LE Diagonal 1 (D1) Extension (with knee extension)	• Dorsiflexion • Inversion • Knee ext. • Hip flexion adduction ext. rot.	• Plantar flexion • Eversion • Knee ext. • Hip extension abduction int. rot.	Turn your heel out and push your foot down and out toward me.

PNF Diagonal Patterns, cont.

Pattern	Start Position	End Position	Commands
LE Diagonal 2 (D2) Flexion (with knee extension)	• Plantar flexion • Inversion • Knee ext. • Hip extension adduction ext. rot.	• Dorsiflexion • Eversion • Knee ext. • Hip flexion abduction int. rot.	Turn your heel out and pull your foot up and out as far as possible.
LE Diagonal 2 (D2) Extension (with knee extension)	• Dorsiflexion • Eversion • Knee ext. • Hip flexion abduction int. rot.	• Plantar flexion • Inversion • Knee ext. • Hip extension adduction ext. rot.	Turn your heel in and push your foot down and in, away from me.

References

Hall, C.M., & Brody, L.T. (2005). *Therapeutic exercise: Moving toward function*. Philadelphia: Lippincott Williams & Wilkins.

Kisner, C., & Colby, L. (2002). *Therapeutic exercise foundations and techniques*. Philadelphia: F.A. Davis.

Voss, D.E., Ionta, M.K., & Myers, B.J. (1985). *Proprioceptive neuromuscular facilitation: Patterns and techniques*. Philadelphia: Harper & Row.

Gait

Deviations/Compensations—Dorsiflexion Dysfunction

Condition: Weak or poorly controlled dorsiflexors

Possible Etiologies: CVA, lumbar radiculopathy, Guillain-Barre, peripheral neuropathy

Interventions: Dorsiflexor strengthening, posterior leaf splint, FES, Marie Foix associated reaction facilitation

Deviation/ Compensation	Description
Drop foot	Excessive plantar flexion during swing
Foot (toe) drag	Dragging of the dorsum of the distal foot/great toe during mid to terminal swing
Foot slap	Rapid, audible plantar flexion at initial contact due to inability of dorsiflexors to eccentrically control plantar flexion
Steppage gait	Characterized by excessive knee and hip flexion during swing to shorten the limb in order to clear the foot
Knee hyperextension	Hyperextension at initial contact as a result of the foot making contact with the supporting surface in plantar flexion, altering the direction of ground resistance forces

continues

Deviations/Compensations——Dorsiflexion Dysfunction, cont.

Vaulting	Deliberate active plantar flexion on the contralateral stance limb in order to facilitate clearance of the swing limb
Hip hiking	Unilateral elevation of the pelvis on the swing side to assist in shortening the limb
Hip circumduction	Combination of flexion/extension and abduction adduction to produce a rotary-type motion; circumduction, hip hiking, and vaulting often combined to facilitate shortening of the swing limb

Deviations/Compensations——Hip Abduction Dysfunction

Condition: Weak or poorly controlled hip flexors

Possible Etiologies: CVA, Guillain-Barre, spinal injury, peripheral neuropathy, deconditioning

Interventions: Abductor strengthening, stair climbing, side stepping

Deviation/ Compensation	Description
Trendelenburg gait	The pelvis on the swing side will drop toward the supporting surface. This is because the contralateral hip abductors are responsible for keeping the pelvic girdle level during the swing phase of gait. This deviation leads to the inability to effectively shorten the limb during swing. Foot clearance may be significantly impaired.
Lateral trunk flexion	Lateral trunk flexion toward the stance side occurs to compensate for the swing side pelvic obliquity that occurs due to insufficient contraction of the stance side abductors.

Deviations/Compensations—Hip Abduction Dysfunction, cont.

Vaulting	Deliberate active plantar flexion on the contralateral stance limb in order to facilitate clearance of the swing limb.
Hip hiking	Unilateral elevation of the pelvis on the swing side to assist in shortening the limb. This maneuver is facilitated through contraction of the quadratus lumborum, latissimus dorsi, and unilateral contraction of erector spinae musculature.
Hip circumduction	Combination of flexion and extension and abduction adduction to produce a rotary-type motion. Circumduction, hip hiking, and vaulting are often combined to facilitate shortening of the swing limb.

Deviations/Compensations—Hip Flexion Dysfunction

Condition: Weak or poorly controlled hip flexors

Possible Etiologies: CVA, Guillain-Barre, peripheral neuropathy, deconditioning

Interventions: Hip flexor strengthening, developmental activities in sidelying and quadruped, stair climbing

Deviation/ Compensation	Description
Excessive hip lateral rotation	The most common rotation deviation is excessive external rotation during early swing. The external rotation positions the limb so that the adductors can pull the limb forward in a pseudoflexion motion.
Hip circumduction	Combination of flexion and extension and abduction adduction to produce a circular-type motion that advances the limb.

continues

Deviations/Compensations—Knee Extension Dysfunction

Condition: Weak or poorly controlled quadriceps

Possible Etiologies: CVA, Guillain-Barre, peripheral neuropathy, deconditioning

Interventions: Quadriceps strengthening, posterior leaf splint, KAFO, NMES, facilitation/control techniques

Deviation/ Compensation	Description
Knee buckling	Rapid, uncontrolled flexion of the knee during stance.
Knee hyperextension or Genu recurvatum	Hyperextension of the knee is most often seen during early stance through midstance. It is often seen as a compensation to prevent buckling.
Trunk flexion	Excessive trunk flexion is often seen during early stance as a complement to knee hyperextension. The trunk flexion is needed to move the center of gravity in front of the knee. If the center of gravity is not shifted, the body weight would remain behind the knee, causing buckling.

Objective Measures and Terms

Term	Description
Gait cycle	The cycle from initial contact on one limb to the next initial contact on the same limb.
Cycle time	The elapsed time, in seconds, required to complete an entire gait cycle.
Step	The movement from swing to initial contact on the same leg.

Objective Measures and Terms, cont.

Term	Description
Step length	The linear distance between two consecutive contralateral foot contacts with the supporting surface. Note: In one gait cycle, there are two step lengths (R-L, L-R).
Stride	One complete gait cycle.
Stride length	The linear distance between two consecutive ipsilateral foot contacts on the walking surface.
Cadence	The number of strides or steps per unit time.
Forward-walking velocity	The rate of linear forward motion of the body. Forward-walking velocity is calculated by measuring the distance between the location of an initial foot contact and a subsequent initial contact and then dividing by the elapsed time.
Heel strike, initial contact, loading, weight acceptance, initial double limb stance	This subdivision of the stance phase of gait initiates when the advancing extremity first contacts the supporting surface. Both lower extremities are supporting the body's weight. Muscular activity and joint placement must be specialized to provide stability and absorb shock.
Midstance, initial single limb stance	This subdivision of stance initiates when the once advancing extremity is now supporting all of the body's weight. This subdivision continues until the contralateral limb makes contact with the supporting surface.
Heel off, preswing, second double limb stance	This subdivision initiates when the contralateral limb has made contact with the supporting surfaces. The limb that initially started out in stance is now preparing for the next phase of gait: swing phase.

continues

Objective Measures and Terms, cont.

Term	Description
Initial swing	This subdivision of swing initiates just as the limb is no longer in contact with the ground. Initial swing is characterized by a period of limb forward acceleration mediated by the hip flexors. This acceleration advances the foot adjacent to the contralateral ankle at that point momentum continues to advance the foot.
Terminal swing, ankle crossing	This subdivision of swing initiates just as the advancing limb passes the contralateral (stance) limb. Rather than accelerating, the limb is now decelerating. Terminal swing ends when the limb makes initial contact with the supporting surface.

Prosthetic Gait Deviations—Transfemoral Amputation

Problem	Potential Causes
Lateral trunk bending over the prosthesis from heel strike to midstance	• weak abductors • abducted socket causing insufficient use of abductors • pain or discomfort along the lateral distal aspect of the femur • short prosthesis
Wide base gait	• proximal medial pain or discomfort • contracted hip abductors • excessively long prosthesis • excessive prosthetic valgus • abducted socket • patient feels insecure
Prosthetic circumduction	• patient flexes the knee insufficiently because of insecurity or fear • manual lock or knee control not allowing knee flexion

Prosthetic Gait Deviations—Transfemoral Amputation, cont.

Problem	Potential Causes
	• inadequate prosthetic suspension • too-small socket • foot set in excessive plantar flexion
Vaulting	• insufficient friction in prosthetic knee • excessive prosthetic length • inadequate suspension • too-small socket • foot set in excessive plantar flexion
Medial prosthetic whip at toe off	• improper alignment of knee bolt in the transverse plane • socket is too tight • weak hip flexors
Prosthetic foot rotation at heel strike	• excessively stiff heel cushion or plantar flexion bumper
Prosthetic foot slap	• excessively soft plantar flexion bumper
Excessive prosthetic heel rise	• insufficient mechanical knee friction • insufficient tension or absence of extension aid • excessively forceful hip flexion
Insufficient prosthetic heel rise	• insufficient mechanical knee friction • too-tight extension aid • absent or worn extension bumper • fear of knee buckling
Uneven step length	• pain or insecurity • hip flexion contracture • insufficient socket flexion • insufficient mechanical knee friction

continues

Prosthetic Gait Deviations—Transfemoral Amputation, cont.

Problem	Potential Causes
Exaggerated lumbar lordosis throughout stance	• hip flexion contracture • insufficient support from anterior socket brim • weak hip extensors • weak abdominal muscles

Prosthetic Gait Deviations—Transtibial Amputation

Problem	Potential Causes
Excessive prosthetic side knee flexion during heel strike	• prosthetic foot set in excessive dorsiflexion • excessive anterior tilt of socket • excessively stiff heel cushion or plantar flexion bumper • flexion contracture
Absent or insufficient knee flexion during heel strike	• prosthetic foot set in excessive plantar flexion • excessively soft heel cushion or plantar flexion bumper • posterior displacement of the socket over the foot • pain at the anterior distal portion of the residual limb
Excessive prosthetic lateral thrust during midstance	• excessive medial placement of the prosthetic foot • excessively abducted socket
Early knee flexion on the prosthetic side during midstance through toe off	• excessive anterior displacement of the socket • excessive posterior placement of prosthetic foot toe break • prosthetic foot set in excessive dorsiflexion • anterior tilt of socket excessively soft dorsiflexor bumper

Prosthetic Gait Deviations—Transtibial Amputation, cont.

Problem	Potential Causes
Delayed knee flexion on the prosthetic side during midstance through toe off	• excessive posterior displacement of the socket • anterior displacement of prosthetic foot toe break • prosthetic foot set in excessive plantar flexion • excessively hard dorsiflexor bumper

References

Lippert, L.S. (2000). *Clinical kinesiology for physical therapist assistants*. Philadelphia: F.A. Davis.

Oatis, C.A. (2004). *Kinesiology: The mechanics and pathomechanics of human movement*. Philadelphia: Lippincott Wiliams & Wilkins.

Prentice, W.E., & Voight, M.I. (2001). *Techniques in musculoskeletal rehabilitation*. New York: McGraw Hill.

5

Pharmacology

Common Intravenous Medications

Trade Name	Generic Name	Therapeutic Action
Activase	Alteplase, Recombinant	Thrombolytic
A-Hydrocort	Hydrocortisone Sodium Succinate	Anti-inflammatory
Ak-Dek	Dexamethasone Sodium Phosphate	Anti-inflammatory
A-MethaPred	Methylprednisolone Sodium Succinate	Anti-inflammatory
APSAC	Anistreplase	Thrombolytic
Astramorph PF	Morphine Sulfate	Narcotic analgesic
AT-III	Antithrombin III	Anticoagulant
Bactrim	Sulfamethoxazole-Trimethoprim	Antibacterial
Bumex	Bumetanide	Diuretic
Buprenex	Buprenorphine Hydrochloride	Narcotic analgesic
C7E3	Abciximab	Anticoagulant
Cathflo Activase	Alteplase, Recombinant	Thrombolytic
Cefotan	Cefotetan Disodium	Antibacterial
Ceptaz	Ceftazidime	Antibacterial
Cipro I.V.	Ciprofloxacin	Antibacterial

continues

Common Intravenous Medications, cont.

Trade Name	Generic Name	Therapeutic Action
Co-Trimoxazole	Sulfamethoxazole-Trimethoprim	Antibacterial
Coumadin	Warfarin Sodium	Anticoagulant
Dalalone	Dexamethasone Sodium Phosphate	Anti-inflammatory
Dalgan	Dezocine	Narcotic analgesic
Decadrol	Dexamethasone Sodium Phosphate	Anti-inflammatory
Decadron	Dexamethasone Sodium Phosphate	Anti-inflammatory
Decadron Phosphate	Dexamethasone Sodium Phosphate	Anti-inflammatory
Decaject	Dexamethasone Sodium Phosphate	Anti-inflammatory
Demadex	Torsemide Injection	Diuretic
Demerol	Meperidine Hydrochloride	Narcotic analgesic
Demerol Hydrochloride	Meperidine Hydrochloride	Narcotic analgesic
Dexasone	Dexamethasone Sodium Phosphate	Anti-inflammatory
Dexone	Dexamethasone Sodium Phosphate	Anti-inflammatory
Dilaudid	Hydromorphone Hydrochloride	Narcotic analgesic
Duramorph	Morphine Sulfate	Narcotic analgesic

Common Intravenous Medications, cont.

Trade Name	Generic Name	Therapeutic Action
Eminase	Anistreplase	Thrombolytic
Floxin I.V.	Ofloxacin	Antibacterial
Fortaz	Ceftazidime	Antibacterial
Furosemide PF	Furosemide	Diuretic
Heparin	Heparin Sodium	Anticoagulant
Hexadrol Phosphate	Dexamethasone Sodium Phosphate	Anti-inflammatory
Hydeltrasol	Prednisolone Sodium Phosphate	Anti-inflammatory
Hydrocortone Phosphate	Hydrocortisone Sodium Phosphate	Anti-inflammatory
Key-Pred SP	Prednisolone Sodium Phosphate	Anti-inflammatory
Lasix	Furosemide	Diuretic
Levo-Dromoran	Levorphanol Tartrate	Narcotic analgesic
Liquaemin Sodium	Heparin Sodium	Anticoagulant
Lysatec	Alteplase, Recombinant	Thrombolytic
Mefoxin	Cefoxitin Sodium	Antibacterial
Numorphan	Oxymorphone Hydrochloride	Narcotic analgesic

Common Intravenous Medications, cont.

Trade Name	Generic Name	Therapeutic Action
Osmitrol	Mannitol	Diuretic
Predicort-RP	Prednisolone Sodium Phosphate	Anti-inflammatory
Prednisolone Phosphate	Prednisolone Sodium Phosphate	Anti-inflammatory
ReoPro	Abciximab	Anticoagulant
Rt-PA	Alteplase, Recombinant	Thrombolytic
Septra	Sulfamethoxazole-Trimethoprim	Antibacterial
Solu-Cortef	Hydrocortisone Sodium Succinate	Anti-inflammatory
Solu-Medrol	Methylprednisolone Sodium Succinate	Anti-inflammatory
Solurex	Dexamethasone Sodium Phosphate	Anti-inflammatory
Tazicef	Ceftazidime	Antibacterial
Tazidime	Ceftazidime	Antibacterial
Thrombate III	Antithrombin III	Anticoagulant
Toradol	Ketorolac Tromethamine	Analgesic (NSAID)
tPA	Alteplase, Recombinant	Thrombolytic

Common Oral Medications, cont.

Brand Name (generic name)	Classification	Description of Action	Adverse Effects
Aldomet (Methyldopa)	Antihypertensive	Affects neurotransmission of the sympathetic nervous system	Initial sedation
Anaprox (Naproxen sodium)	Nonsteroidal anti-inflammatory	Provides pain relief by inhibiting production of prostaglandins	Upper respiratory infection Diarrhea Stomach cramps Heartburn
Ansaid (Flurbiprofen)	Nonsteroidal anti-inflammatory	Provides pain relief by inhibiting production of prostaglandins	Abdominal pain Diarrhea Indigestion Nausea
Bextra (Valdecoxib) [Removed from market]	Nonsteroidal anti-inflammatory COX-2 Inhibitor	Provides pain relief by inhibiting production of prostaglandins associated with the inflammatory process while sparing the production	Upper respiratory infection Diarrhea Stomach cramps Heartburn

continues

Common Oral Medications, cont.

Brand Name (generic name)	Classification	Description of Action	Adverse Effects
Bextra, (con't)		of physiological protective prostaglandins	Cardiovascular risks
Capoten (Captopril)	Angiotensin converting enzyme (ACE) inhibitor Antihypertensive	Decreases salt and water retention	Itching Loss of taste Rash Hypotension
Cardizem (Diltiazem hydrochloride)	Calcium-channel blocker Antihypertensive Antiangina pectoris	Dilates blood vessels and slows heart	Bradycardia Fatigue Headache Weakness
Celebrex (Celecoxib)	Nonsteroidal anti-inflammatory COX-2 Inhibitor	Provides pain relief by inhibiting production of prostaglandins associated with the inflammatory process while sparing the production of physiological protective prostaglandins	Upper respiratory infection Diarrhea Stomach cramps Heartburn Cardiovascular risks

Common Oral Medications, cont.

Brand Name (generic name)	Classification	Description of Action	Adverse Effects
Clinoril (Sulindac)	Nonsteroidal anti-inflammatory	Provides pain relief by inhibiting production of prostaglandins	Abdominal pain Diarrhea Indigestion Nausea
Darvocet-N (Propoxyphene napsylate)	Narcotic analgesic	Relieves pain through action on the central nervous system	Drowsiness Dizziness Nausea Vomiting
Daypro (Oxaprozin)	Nonsteroidal anti-inflammatory	Provides pain relief by inhibiting production of prostaglandins	Abdominal pain Diarrhea Indigestion Nausea

continues

Common Oral Medications, cont.

Brand Name (generic name)	Classification	Description of Action	Adverse Effects
Decadron (Dexamethasone)	Corticosteroid anti-inflammatory	Mimics steroid hormones that affect the body's chemical reactions to stress	Weight gain Hypertension Facial hair Hyperglycemia Headache Increased appetite
Demerol (Meperidine hydrochloride)	Narcotic analgesic	Relieves pain through action on the central nervous system.	Drowsiness Dizziness Nausea Vomiting
Depakote (Valproic acid)	Antiseizure	Changes chemical balances in the brain that decreases neuronal excitability	Abdominal pain Altered thinking Bronchitis Depression Drowsiness

Common Oral Medications, cont.

Brand Name (generic name)	Classification	Description of Action	Adverse Effects
DiaBeta (Glyburide)	Antidiabetic	Stimulates the pancreas to produce more insulin and boosts insulin action	Bloating Heartburn Nausea
Diabinese (Chlorpropamide)	Antidiabetic	Stimulates the pancreas to produce more insulin and boosts insulin action	Diarrhea Hunger Itching Nausea
Dilantin (Phenytoin sodium)	Antiseizure	Changes chemical balances in the brain that decreases neuronal excitability	Decreased coordination Confusion Slurred speech
Dolobid (Diflunisal)	Nonsteroidal anti-inflammatory	Provides pain relief by inhibiting production of prostaglandins	Abdominal pain Diarrhea Constipation Nausea Dizziness Tinnitus

continues

Common Oral Medications, cont.

Brand Name (generic name)	Classification	Description of Action	Adverse Effects
Elavil (Amitriptyline hydrochloride)	Antidepression	Stimulates the central nervous system resulting in mood elevation	Blurred vision Bone marrow depression Dry mouth Constipation
Embrel (Etanercept)	Rheumatoid Arthritis management	Blocks the action of protein factor active in rheumatoid arthritis	Abdominal pain Infections
Feldene (Piroxicam)	Nonsteroidal anti-inflammatory	Provides pain relief by inhibiting production of prostaglandins	Abdominal pain Diarrhea Constipation Nausea Fluid retention Tinnitus Stomach ulcer

Common Oral Medications, cont.

Brand Name (generic name)	Classification	Description of Action	Adverse Effects
Fioricet (Butalbital)	Nonnarcotic analgesic Muscle relaxant	Provides pain release and relaxant effects by combining a sedative, nonaspirin pain reliever, and caffeine	Abdominal pain Dizziness Drowsiness Nausea
Flexeril (cyclobezaprine hydrochloride)	Muscle relaxant	Provides muscle relaxation by modifying CNS influence on skeletal muscle	Dizziness Drowsiness Dry mouth
Fosamax (Alendronate sodium)	Antiresorptive for osteoporosis management and prevention	Slows bone loss	Abdominal pain Acid regurgitation Joint pain Indigestion
Glucophage (Metformin hydrochloride)	Antidiabetic	Decreases the body's production of glucose and facilitates insulin response	Abdominal pain Diarrhea Indigestion

continues

Common Oral Medications, cont.

Brand Name (generic name)	Classification	Description of Action	Adverse Effects
Glucotrol (Glipizide)	Antidiabetic	Stimulates the pancreas to produce more insulin and boosts insulin action	Constipation Diarrhea Dizziness Headache Nervousness
Glucovance (Glyburide and Metformin)	Antidiabetic	Stimulates pancreas production and facilitates insulin response	Cold sweats Diarrhea Headache Hunger Nausea
Inderal (Propanolol hydrochloride)	Beta-blocker Antihypertensive Antiangina	Interferes with adrenaline action resulting in the slowing of the heart rate	Abdominal cramps CHF Depression Fatigue

Common Oral Medications, cont.

Brand Name (generic name)	Classification	Description of Action	Adverse Effects
Indocin (Indomethacin)	Nonsteroidal anti-inflammatory	Provides pain relief by inhibiting production of prostaglandins	Abdominal pain Diarrhea Constipation Nausea Tinnitus
Lanoxin (Digoxin)	CHF management Antiarrhythmia	Improves the strength and efficiency of the heartbeat	Apathy Blurred vision Diarrhea Dizziness
Lasix (Furosemide)	Diuretic Antihypertensive CHF management	Affects kidney function resulting in the elimination of excess fluid	Anemia Constipation Hypokalemia Muscle spasms

continues

Common Oral Medications, cont.

Brand Name (generic name)	Classification	Description of Action	Adverse Effects
Lodine (Etodolac)	Nonsteroidal anti-inflammatory	Provides pain relief by inhibiting production of prostaglandins	Abdominal pain Diarrhea Constipation Nausea Tinnitus
Lopressor (Metoprolol tartrate)	Beta-blocker Antihypertensive Antiangina	Interferes with adrenaline action resulting in the slowing of the heart rate	Depression Diarrhea Dizziness SOB Bradycardia
Medrol (Methylprednisolone)	Corticosteroid anti-inflammatory	Mimics steroid hormones that affect the body's chemical reactions to stress	Weight gain Hypertension Facial hair Hyperglycemia

Common Oral Medications, cont.

Brand Name (generic name)	Classification	Description of Action	Adverse Effects
Medrol (cont.)			Headache Increased appetite
Motrin (Ibuprofen)	Nonsteroidal anti-inflammatory	Provides pain relief by inhibiting production of prostaglandins	Abdominal pain Diarrhea Constipation Nausea Tinnitus
Naprosyn (Naproxen)	Nonsteroidal anti-inflammatory	Provides pain relief by inhibiting production of prostaglandins	Abdominal pain Diarrhea Constipation Nausea Tinnitus
Orudis (Ketoprofen)	Nonsteroidal anti-inflammatory	Provides pain relief by inhibiting production of prostaglandins	Abdominal pain Kidney function impairment Diarrhea Constipation

continues

Common Oral Medications, cont.

Brand Name (generic name)	Classification	Description of Action	Adverse Effects
Oxycontin (Oxycodone hydrochloride)	Narcotic analgesic	Relieves pain through action on the central nervous system	Constipation Drowsiness Dizziness Nausea Vomiting
Parafon Forte (Chlorzoxazone)	Muscle relaxant	Relaxes muscle by affecting spinal and subcortical neurons inhibiting multisynaptic reflex arcs	Mild drowsiness
Percocet (Acetaminophen, Oxycodone hydrochloride)	Narcotic analgesic Antipyretic	Reduces pain and fever	Dizziness Nausea Vomiting

Common Oral Medications, cont.

Brand Name (generic name)	Classification	Description of Action	Adverse Effects
Relafen (Nabumetone)	Nonsteroidal anti-inflammatory	Provides pain relief by inhibiting production of prostaglandins	Abdominal pain Diarrhea Constipation Nausea Tinnitus
Robaxin (Methocarbamol)	Muscle relaxant	Exact mechanism of action is not known, however, relaxation achieved through nervous system mediation	Abnormal taste Blurred vision Confusion Dizziness Drowsiness
Sinemet (Carbidopa, Levodopa)	Anti-Parkinson's	Facilitates the production of dopamine	Confusion Hallucinations Nausea

continues

Common Oral Medications, cont.

Brand Name (generic name)	Classification	Description of Action	Adverse Effects
Tegretol (Carbamazepine)	Antiseizure	Affects sodium shifts in the brain and helps stabilize neuronal activity	Dizziness Drowsiness Nausea Unsteadiness
Theo-Dur (Theophylline)	Broncho-dilator	Relaxes smooth muscle lining airways	Convulsions Diarrhea Arrhythmia Excitability
Ultracet (Tramadol hydrochloride, Acetaminophen)	Analgesic	Combines narcotic and nonnarcotic agents for pain relief	Constipation Increased sweating Drowsiness

Common Oral Medications, cont.

Brand Name (generic name)	Classification	Description of Action	Adverse Effects
Ultram (Tramadol hydrochloride)	Narcotic analgesic	Binds with opioid pain receptors	Agitation Anxiety Bloating Drowsiness Dizziness
Valium (Diazepam)	Antianxiety Muscle relaxant	Works directly at emotion centers in the brain	Anxiety Drowsiness Fatigue Dizziness
Vicodin (Hydrocodone bitartrate, Acetaminophen)	Analgesic	Combines narcotic and nonnarcotic agents for pain relief	Dizziness Nausea Sedation

Common Oral Medications, cont.

Brand Name (generic name)	Classification	Description of Action	Adverse Effects
Vioxx (Rofecoxib) [removed from market]	Nonsteroidal anti-inflammatory COX-2 Inhibitor	Provides pain relief by inhibiting production of prostaglandins associated with the inflammatory process while sparing the production of physiological protective prostaglandins	Upper respiratory infection Diarrhea Stomach cramps Heartburn Cardiovascular risks
Voltaren (Diclofenac sodium)	Nonsteroidal anti-inflammatory	Provides pain relief by inhibiting production of prostaglandins	Abdominal pain Diarrhea Constipation Nausea Tinnitus
Zanaflex (Tizanidine)	Muscle relaxant Antispasticity	Inhibits CNS motor pathways	Abnormal movements Blurred vision Constipation Dizziness

Listing of Oral Medications by Classification

Classification	Brand Name (Generic Name)
Antidiabetic	• Diabeta (Glyburide)
	• Diabinese (Chlorpropamide)
	• Glucophage (Metformin hydrochloride)
	• Glucotrol (Glipizide)
	• Glucovance (Glyburide and Metformin)
Antihypertensive	• Aldomet (Methyldopa)
	• Capoten ((Captopril)
	• Cardizem (Diltiazen hydrochloride)
	• Inderal (Propanolol hydrochloride)
	• Lasix (Furosemide)
	• Lopressor (Metoprolol tartrate)
Antiseizure	• Depakote (Valproic acid)
	• Dilantin (Phenytoin sodium)
	• Tegretol (Carbamazepine)
Muscle Relaxant	• Fiorcet (Butalbital)
	• Flexeril (Cyclobezaprine hydrochloride)
	• Parafon Forte (Chlorzoxazone)
	• Robaxin (Methocarbamol)
	• Valium (Diazepam)
	• Zanaflex (Tizanidine)
Narcotic Analgesic	• Darvocet-N (Propoxyphene napsylate)
	• Demerol (Meperidine hydrochloride)
	• Oxycontin (Oxycodone hydrochloride)
	• Percocet (Acetaminophen, Oxycodone hydrochloride)
	• Ultram (Tramadol hydrochloride)
Nonsteroidal Anti-inflammatory	• Anaprox (Naproxen sodium)
	• Ansaid (Flurbiprofen)
	• Bextra (Valdecoxib); removed from market
	• Celebrex (Celecoxib)
	• Clinoril (Sulindac)

Listing of Oral Medications by Classification, cont.

Classification	Brand Name (Generic Name)
Nonsteroidal Anti-inflammatory (con't)	• Daypro (Oxaprozin)
	• Dolobid (Diflunisal)
	• Feldene (Piroxicam)
	• Indocin (Indomethacin)
	• Lodine (Etodolac)
	• Motrin (Ibuprofen)
	• Naprosyn (Naproxen)
	• Orudis (Ketoprofen)
	• Relafen (Nabumetone)
	• Vioxx (Rofecoxib); removed from market
	• Voltaren (Diclofenac sodium)

References

Gahart, B. (2003). *Intravenous medications: A handbook for nurses and allied health professionals*. St. Louis, MO: Mosby.

Thompson Healthcare. (2005). *PDRhealth*. Retrieved October 25, 2005, from www.pdrhealth.com.

Common Pathologies

Adhesive Capsulitis of the Shoulder

Classification   Adhesive capsulitis is also known as frozen shoulder in which adhesions and capsular restrictions occur in the fold of the capsule. Adhesive capsulitis may be primary or secondary. Primary adhesive capsulitis has no known cause. Secondary adhesive capsulitis is the result of a traumatic incident such as a fracture or other pathological condition (i.e., rotator cuff tear).

Manifestations   Adhesive capsulitis may be subdivided into three phases: freezing phase, frozen phase, and thawing phase.

In the **freezing phase,** the patient may experience pain, muscle guarding with shoulder external rotation and abduction. The patient may have pain at rest or with activity. This phase may last 2 to 9 months.

In the **frozen phase,** limitations in ROM and joint play occur. Limitations are initially in external rotation and abduction followed by flexion and internal rotation. The patient may complain of pain at the end of the ROM. This is considered the inflammatory phase. As the phase progresses, the

continues

Adhesive Capsulitis of the Shoulder, cont.

patient may experience muscle atrophy of the deltoid, biceps, and triceps muscles. The patient may have tenderness upon palpation at the anterior joint capsule. This phase may last 4 to 9 months.

In the **thawing phase,** the patient may have no complaints of pain but have capsular restrictions. This phase may last 2 to 24 months.

Medical Management	Adhesive capsulitis is diagnosed through physical examination. NSAIDS are prescribed to treat associated inflammation and pain. Physicians often prescribe physical therapy. In cases where there is a lack of progress, surgery may be indicated to treat an underlying condition or a manipulation may be performed to improve motion.
Physical Therapy Goals	Patients are typically treated in outpatient facilities. Goals include decreasing inflammation and improving ROM and strength.
	Improving the patient's ability to perform overhead, dressing, and other functional activities are common goals.
Effective PT Interventions	Physical therapy treatment includes superficial heat, ultrasound, ice, and electrical stimulation depending on symptoms and extent of pathology.
	Modalities are used to relieve pain and inflammation and to prepare the shoulder for mobilization and stretching.
	During the acute phase, gentle mobilization (Grade I or II) techniques may be used in the direction of limitations. Passive ROM, Codman's exercise, and muscle-setting exercises are also used when the patient is in an acute phase.

Adhesive Capsulitis of the Shoulder, cont.

Patients progress to active assistive and active ROM in the pain-free range. Gentle self-stretching and passive stretching is performed to improve ROM once pain is better managed.

Effective treatment incorporates scapular mobilization and glenohumeral mobilization and appropriate strengthening exercises at all phases. Maintenance of strength and ROM at the wrist may also be addressed.

Precautions   Aggressive stretching should be avoided in the acute phase of treatment. Manual interventions and exercise dosages should be decreased if pain increases after treatment.

Amputation—Transfemoral/Above the Knee

Classification   Transfemoral amputation involves the surgical removal of the lower extremity from the mid to proximal third of the femur. Amputations are most frequently performed secondary to circulation impairment and resulting sepsis in severe peripheral vascular disorders. In North America, complications of diabetes mellitus account for the vast majority of amputations.

Manifestations   Presurgical manifestations often include weak or absent peripheral pulses, recurrent open wounds with infection, and moderate to severe pain. Postsurgical manifestations include residual limb or phantom pain, edema, muscle weakness, and gait disturbance.

Medical Management   Postsurgical management includes the use of antibiotics, NSAIDS, and pain medication. Early rehabilitation intervention is crucial to maximize function.

continues

Amputation—Transfemoral/Above the Knee, cont.

Physical Therapy Goals	Patient education related to appropriate positioning (no pillows under residual limb, avoidance of sidelying) is a crucial goal in order to avoid the development of hip contractures.
	Early movement and strengthening of hip musculature is important. Shaping and edema management of the residual limb is critical for ultimate prosthetic fit.
	Other goals include facilitation and maintenance of balance, increasing muscle strength in all extremities, facilitation of weight shifting, and ADL (crutch/walker, transfers, etc.).
Effective PT Interventions	Given the patient's complete reliance on the noninvolved lower extremity and both upper extremities to move from sit to stand, appropriate strengthening of the musculature of these extremities is a crucial part of postamputation rehabilitation.
	SLR, terminal knee extension, full arc quadriceps, hip abduction, and adduction activities, as well as general UE strengthening with emphasis placed on the shoulder depressors enhance muscle strength for transfer training.
	Sit-to-stand transfer activities from variable seat heights and depths are effective. Use of large therapeutic ball for weight shifting to involved side and general balance activities in standing are helpful.
	Trunk rotation activities in sitting and standing facilitate more efficient future gait patterns.
	Use of ace wraps and shrinkers for edema control and residual limb shaping are effective. However, careful comparative circumferential assessments should be performed to gauge progress.

Amputation—Transfemoral/Above the Knee, cont.

Manual resistive strengthening of residual limb hip musculature will facilitate a more efficient gait and better prosthetic control. Manual resistive exercise, though less objective, may be more effective given the shorter lever arm of the residual limb.

Precautions   Monitor vascular status of uninvolved extremity. Monitor residual limb skin condition. Monitor suture line. Monitor pain symptoms.

Amputation—Transtibial/Below the Knee

Classification   Transtibial amputation involves the surgical removal of the lower extremity from the proximal third of the tibia. Performed most often secondary to circulation impairment and resulting sepsis in severe peripheral vascular disorders. In North America, complications of diabetes mellitus accounts for the vast majority of amputations.

Manifestations   Presurgical manifestations often include weak or absent peripheral pulses, recurrent open wounds with infection, and moderate to severe pain. Postsurgical manifestations include residual limb or phantom pain, edema, muscle weakness, and gait disturbance.

Medical Management   Postsurgical management includes the use of antibiotics, NSAIDS, and pain medication. Early rehabilitation intervention is crucial to maximize function.

Physical Therapy Goals   Patient education related to appropriate positioning (no pillows under residual limb, avoidance of sidelying) is a crucial goal in order to avoid the development of hip and knee flexion contractures.

continues

Amputation—Transtibial/Below the Knee, cont.

Early movement and strengthening of bilateral hip and knee musculature is important.

Shaping and edema management of residual limb is critical for ultimate prosthetic fit.

Other goals include facilitation and maintenance of balance, increase muscle strength in all extremities, facilitation of weight shifting, and ADL (crutch/walker, transfers, etc.).

Effective PT Interventions

Given the significantly reduced lever arm, manually resisted residual limb strengthening activities, though less objective, are effective.

Sit-to-stand transfer activities from variable seat heights and depths are useful.

Pre- and postprosthetic weight shifting to the involved side and general balance activities in standing are helpful.

Trunk rotation activities in sitting and standing facilitate more efficient future gait patterns.

Use of ace wraps and shrinkers for edema control and residual limb shaping are effective. However, careful comparative circumferential assessments should be performed to gauge progress.

Precautions

Monitor vascular status of uninvolved extremity. Monitor residual limb skin condition. Monitor suture line. Monitor pain symptoms.

Amyotrophic Lateral Sclerosis

Classification

Amyotrophic lateral sclerosis (ALS) is an adult-onset progressive motor neuron disease. Its etiology is unknown. The disease is characterized by scarring of motor neurons in the lateral aspect of the spinal cord, brain stem, and cerebral cortex. Also known as Lou Gehrig's disease.

Amyotrophic Lateral Sclerosis, cont.

Manifestations Clinical manifestations may vary depending on whether upper motor neuron or lower motor neurons are initially involved.

Lower motor neuron involvement includes initial asymmetric distal weakness with progression to other muscles of that limb. This gradually progresses to increased weakness of extensor musculature, especially in the cervical spine and upper extremities. Impaired control of chewing, swallowing, and phonation is also noted. Progressive wasting and atrophy of skeletal muscles is noted.

Upper motor neuron symptoms include impaired dexterity, spasticity, loss of strength/control, and hyperactive reflexes.

Ultimately, both upper and lower motor neurons are involved.

Medical Management ALS is usually diagnosed based upon EMG and clinical findings. There is no known cure for ALS.

Some drugs (e.g., riluzole) may be effective in slowing the progression. Other medications are used for symptomatic relief of spasticity, drooling, and other manifestations.

Nutritional intake modifications may be required as chewing and swallowing difficulties progress.

Physical Therapy Goals PT management of ALS will often initially occur on an outpatient or home care basis.

Initial goals are based upon maintaining the patient's functional status. In early onset cases, goals include the maintenance of strength and range of motion.

continues

Amyotrophic Lateral Sclerosis, cont.

As symptoms progress, goals include appropriate training of use of assistive devices, cautious strengthening of muscles graded F+ or higher, appropriate orthotic support, pulmonary hygiene, integument monitoring, wheelchair modifications, etc.

Effective PT Interventions   Manually resisted exercises allow for assessment of strength and fatigue. Though these exercises are less objective, the variable resistance nature may provide a more strenuous exercise without causing excessive fatigue.

Passive, active, and active-assisted range of motion activities for all extremities should be taught and performed regularly.

Wand activities, overhead pulley activities, stationary bicycle/restorator combine strengthening and ROM and are effective, especially when managing fatigue.

Use of elastic resistance devices is helpful for home exercise regimens.

Precautions   Avoid excessive fatigue during therapeutic exercise. Respiratory status should be assessed frequently. Skin condition in areas of increased pressure should be carefully monitored.

Anterior Cruciate Ligament Injuries

Classification   The anterior cruciate ligament (ACL) is the most commonly torn knee ligament. The ACL prevents the tibia from moving too far forward and prevents hyperextension of the knee joint. Injuries to the ACL usually result from twisting movements, sidestepping, pivoting, landing from a jump, or blows to the lateral side of the knee. It should be noted that injuries to the knee commonly result in injury to multiple accessory structures.

Anterior Cruciate Ligament Injuries, cont.

Manifestations   ACL injuries occur in varying degrees. As a result, impairments will vary in severity. Immediately following injury to the ACL, the knee will be swollen and the patient may not be able to weight bear secondary to pain. Following this acute stage, patients will complain of pain, instability, and difficulty performing pivoting movements.

Medical Management   Medical management of an ACL tear is dependent on the extent of the injury, degree of instability, and the patient's activity level. Patients are diagnosed through physical exam, including a number of special tests and MRI.

Patients who are not going to be involved in sports may be able to function normally with a damaged ACL. Conservative management of ACL tears includes a period of physical therapy for range of motion and strengthening and possible bracing.

More active patients will require surgical reconstruction or repair of the ACL. Reconstruction surgery may be extra- or intraarticular. Extraarticular reconstruction involves surgery to other areas of the knee to compensate for the insufficient ACL (e.g., tightening of the iliotibial band to prevent excessive excursion of the knee).

Intraarticular reconstruction involves tissue grafting. Part of the patella or hamstring tendon or donor tissue from a cadaver may be used as a graft. Surgery may be done by an open procedure or arthroscopically. In rare instances, the ACL may be repaired. However, due to the decreased vascularity, repairs are not often successful.

continues

Anterior Cruciate Ligament Injuries, cont.

Physical Therapy Goals

Physical therapy will vary depending on whether the patient is being treated conservatively. Despite changes in time frame, physical therapy goals for surgical and nonsurgical will be to regain ROM, strength, balance control, knee stability, and to improve functional activities and gait.

Effective PT Interventions

Nonsurgical management focuses on decreasing pain and edema through cold modalities, electrical stimulation, and compression. Exercises should include passive, active assistive and active range of motion (AROM) within the pain-free range and quadriceps setting exercises.

As the patient moves out of the acute phase, joint mobility and strengthening is initiated. Exercises include AROM exercises, patella mobilization, cycling on a stationary bicycle, straight leg raises, open chain resistive exercises, and closed chain activities to improve stability. Closed chain exercises may include partial squats, leg press, heel raises, and balance and gait training.

Postsurgical management is often directed by a specific protocol. There are several ACL rehabilitation protocols. A specific protocol is chosen by the physician dependent upon the type of surgery, relative conservatism, and other factors. Effective rehabilitation requires strict adherence to the chosen protocol.

Initially, outpatient therapy typically consists of ambulation training with crutches, muscle-setting exercises, passive range of motion (PROM), active assistive range of motion (AAROM), ankle pumps, and edema control.

Anterior Cruciate Ligament Injuries, cont.

Muscle setting exercises may include quadriceps and hamstring sets. Straight-leg raises (SLR) in supine may also be initiated.

Ice and electrical stimulation may be used for edema and pain control. Patients may then be progressed according to protocol and surgeon's prescription.

Patients are progressed to multiangle isometric exercises and open chain exercises (i.e., knee extension; range 90° to 40°), and active SLR in supine, prone, and sidelying.

As the patient continues to progress and is able to fully weight bear, closed chain activities may be initiated (i.e., single leg stance activities, balance or rocker board and stabilization exercises, and balance activities). Endurance training may include exercise on a stationary bicycle and aquatic exercises.

Increasing weight is placed on the affected limb during flexion, extension, abduction, and adduction exercises. Closed chain exercises increase in intensity to include plyometric activities, once cleared by the surgeon.

Running, hopping, and jumping drills are performed near the end of the rehabilitation process to ensure joint stability and prepare the patient to resume sporting or full functional activities.

Precautions   Resistive open chain knee extension exercise from 60° to 0° and closed chain exercises between 60° and 90° should be avoided. During closed chain exercises, the knee should not come forward over the toes.

continues

Carpal Tunnel Syndrome

Classification

Carpal tunnel syndrome (CTS) is a repetitive-use injury of the wrist. It is caused from compression of the median nerve as a result of flexor tenosynovitis within the carpal tunnel. The etiology of CTS is often due to occupational activities such as repetitive or forceful gripping. CTS may also be seen in people with rheumatoid tenosynovitis, edema, pregnancy, and hypothyroidism.

Manifestations

Initially, clinical manifestations include pain, numbness, and tingling along the median nerve distribution. Patients may complain of pain at the wrist, forearm, or first three fingers.

As CTS progresses, patients may experience pain radiating to the arm and shoulder. Sensory changes occur at the first four and one half fingers on the palmer surface and the distal fingers on the dorsal surface of the hand.

Weakness in the hand may also occur as CTS progresses. Besides impairment in performing occupational activities, patients complain of difficulty driving and holding a newspaper.

Medical Management

Diagnosis of CTS is made through physical examination and clinical tests including Phalen's or Tinel's test. Treatment for CTS may take an operative or nonoperative approach.

Nonoperative management may include splinting, physical therapy, and medication. Frequently prescribed medications include NSAIDS, corticosteroids, lidocaine, and diuretics.

Surgical management includes open or endoscopic release. In the open release surgery, the carpal tunnel ligament is cut to increase tunnel space. In

Carpal Tunnel Syndrome, cont.

the endoscopic release, the carpal tunnel ligament is also cut but without using an invasive procedure which can lead to faster recovery.

Physical Therapy Goals

Patients with CTS are seen on an outpatient basis. Physical therapy goals include pain management and stretching and strengthening, as well as patient education. Progressions toward these goals will vary depending on whether or not management is operative or nonoperative.

Effective PT Interventions

Management of nonoperative patients includes splinting, patient education, workplace modification, joint mobilization of the carpals, tendon gliding, gentle strengthening, and endurance exercises.

Patient education should include suggestions for modifications of aggravating activities. Initial exercises may include multiangle muscle-setting exercises with progression to strengthening and endurance activities for the forearm, wrist, and hand. Elastic resistive devices, small dumbbells, wrist weights, and therapeutic putty are effective for strengthening.

Modalities may also be used to control pain and decrease inflammation including cold, heat, electrical stimulation, and low-level laser (approved in 2003 in the United States for CTS).

For postoperative patients, physical therapy should follow the individual surgeon's protocols. Initial treatment usually involves pain and edema control. Tendon gliding and AROM exercises for wrist extension, radial/ulnar deviation, and finger motions can be done initially.

continues

Carpal Tunnel Syndrome, cont.

As patients recover, care should be taken to mobilize the scar, progress strengthening exercises, and begin stretching activities. Patients are educated on how to look for signs of inflammation and how to modify activities during the healing process.

Precautions   Surgical patients may have specific postoperative precautions. One example would be no active finger flexion with wrist flexion for the first 10 days. Adherence to postsurgical rehabilitation protocol is crucial.

Cerebral Vascular Accident—General Information

Classifications   Cerebral vascular accident (CVA) (also known as a stroke) is a sudden loss or compromise of oxygen and nutrients to the brain with resulting tissue damage. This loss comes about due to pathologic changes in the heart and/or vascular tree providing blood to the brain. Because central nervous system neurons do not regenerate effectively, tissue damage persists, causing long-term signs and symptoms.

Manifestations   Clinical manifestations vary depending upon the type of stroke (hemorrhagic vs. ischemic) and location. Generally, clinical manifestations include change in muscle tone, alteration in cognitive functions, perceptual impairment, and impaired motor control. The most classic sign is hemiplegia or hemiparesis.

Medical Management   Sound diagnosis is the hallmark of CVA management. The use of CT and MRI imaging techniques provide for specific determination of location, type, and extent of lesions.

Cerebral Vascular Accident—General Information, cont.

Medical treatment includes the management of precipitating factors including hypertensive and cardiac conditions. The use of effective agents to dissolve thromboses is increasing.

Preventive measures are perhaps the best medical management. Preventive measures include the use of cholesterol and blood pressure–lowering agents.

Physical Therapy Goals

Given the variability in the signs and symptoms, physical therapy goals must be carefully tailored to the individual patient. General physical therapy goals include the normalization of muscle tone, facilitation of normal and the inhibition of abnormal motor patterns, facilitation of appropriate compensatory motor strategies, and functional enhancement of gait and ADL.

Effective PT Interventions

There are several approaches to the PT management of CVA. The clinician is best guided by techniques that seem most effective for the patient. This may include employing strategies from schools including Rood, Brunnstrom, and Bobath.

Other strategies revolve around the goal of maximizing function in gait and functional activities. Traditional therapeutic exercise and electrical stimulation may be used to activate and strengthen muscles still under adequate central control.

Cerebral Vascular Accident—Common Terms and Symptoms Descriptions

Abulia

Abulia is the loss or impairment of the ability to carry out voluntary actions or to make decisions. It is also characterized by a reduction or delay in speech and emotional action. Abulia is associated with anterior cerebral artery syndrome.   *continues*

Cerebral Vascular Accident—Common Terms and Symptoms Descriptions, cont.

Agnosia	Agnosia is the loss or impairment of the ability to recognize or comprehend sensory stimuli. Agnosia includes impairment of tactile; the inability to recognize objects by touch or sight; the inability to recognize objects by sight or color; the inability to recognize colors or sounds; the inability to recognize words or music.
Agraphia	Agraphia is the loss or impairment of the ability to write.
Alexia	Alexia is the loss or impairment of the ability to read.
Anomia	Anomia is a form of aphasia characterized by loss or impairment of ability to name objects that are seen, heard, or felt.
Aphasia	Aphasia is a general loss or impairment of communication.
Expressive	Deficits in speech production or language output characterize this aphasia.
Receptive	Deficits in comprehension of written or spoken communication characterize this aphasia.
Global	Deficits in all aspects of communication characterize this aphasia.
Broca's Aphasia	This expressive aphasia may result with compromise to the left frontal lobe region of the brain. It is characterized by difficulty forming meaningful phrases. People with this aphasia frequently speak in short phrases omitting small words such as and, is, and for. Because this is an expressive aphasia, those suffering with Broca's aphasia often become

Cerebral Vascular Accident—Common Terms and Symptoms Descriptions, cont.

	very frustrated with their inability to communicate effectively.
Wernicke's Aphasia	This global aphasia may result with compromise to the left temporal lobe. It is characterized by individuals forming long sentences that have no meaning. Individuals may use unnecessary words and may even create their own words.
Apraxia	Apraxia is the loss or impairment in the performance of skilled or purposeful movement. It is typically thought of as a motor-planning deficit.
Ataxia	Ataxia is the loss or impairment of the ability to coordinate muscle activity. Ataxia leads to jerky, discontinuous, and inefficient motion.
Dizziness	Dizziness is a symptom described by patients as the feeling of faintness, lightheadedness, and/or the apparent spinning of objects in the environment.
Dysarthria	Dysarthria refers to a general disruption in speech and language resulting from paralysis, incoordination, or spasticity of muscles of phonation.
Dysdiadochokinesia	Dysdiadochokinesia is the inability to perform rapidly alternating movements.
Dysmetria	Dysmetria is a specific type of ataxia characterized by impairment in controlling the speed, distance, and power of motor acts.
Dysphagia	Dysphagia is difficulty in swallowing
Hemianesthesia	Hemianesthesia is the loss or impairment of sensation on one side of the body.

continues

Cerebral Vascular Accident—Common Terms and Symptoms Descriptions, cont.

Hemiparesis	Hemiparesis refers to impaired motor control on one side of the body.
Hemiplegia	Hemiplegia is characterized by paralysis of one side of the body.
Hoarseness	Hoarseness is a voice quality that is rough and/or harsh.
Homonymous Hemianopsia	Homonymous hemianopsia is the loss of vision in one half of the visual field in both eyes.
Intracerebral Hemorrhage (ICH)	An intracerebral hemorrhage is bleeding from arteries into brain tissue. ICH type strokes are typically the most serious.
Ischemic Stroke	An ischemic stroke is a CVA that comes about due to a blockage of arterial blood to brain tissue. An ischemic stroke is caused by either a static thrombosis or an embolus that has lodged in an artery.
Neglect	Neglect is a clinical manifestation of CVA characterized by significant patient inattention to the affected side.
Nystagmus	Nystagmus is a rhythmic oscillation of the eyeballs.
Paresthesias	Paresthesias are abnormal sensations that include burning, tingling, prickling, etc.
Ptosis	Ptosis (pronounced *tosis*) is a drooping of the eyelid.
Vertigo	Vertigo is a symptom described by patients as the feeling of faintness or light headedness. Vertigo may be distinguished from dizziness by the report of spinning of the patient's internal environment rather than the apparent spinning of objects in the external environment.

Cerebral Vascular Accident—Clinical Syndromes

Neurologists often describe cerebral vascular accidents by the major artery involved. Because these arteries provide nutrients to specific areas, the result is somewhat stereotypical syndromes.

Middle Cerebral Artery Syndrome If this artery is occluded at its stem, symptoms may include contralateral hemiparesis and hemianesthesia and global aphasia. Partial occlusion symptoms may include impaired contralateral upper extremity motor control, facial droop with motor apraxia, sensory disturbance, and Wernicke's aphasia.

Anterior Cerebral Artery Syndrome This is a rare syndrome. Symptoms may include contralateral hemiparesis with the lower extremity more involved than the upper extremity.

Posterior Cerebral Artery Syndrome Symptoms may include sensation disturbances of pain, proprioception, temperature, and touch. Hemiplegia and involvement of cranial nerve III (oculomotor) may occur. Homonymous hemianopsia, memory disturbance, alexia, and agraphia may also occur.

Vertebral and Posterior Inferior Cerebellar Artery Syndrome Symptoms may include contralateral upper and lower extremity hemiparesis, dysphagia, vertigo, ptosis, paresthesias of face and limbs, and gait unsteadiness.

Basilar Artery Syndrome Symptoms are characterized by cranial nerve involvement.

Superior Cerebellar Syndrome Symptoms may include ataxia, nausea, and dysarthria.

Anterior Inferior Cerebellar Artery Syndrome Symptoms may include ipsilateral deafness, vertigo, nystagmus, and facial weakness.

Lacunar Syndrome Lacunar occlusions are small infarcts at the ends of arteries. They are often seen in deep brain tissue

continues

Cerebral Vascular Accident—Clinical Syndromes, cont.

including the basal ganglia, internal capsule, and pons. Lacunar infarcts may present as diffuse, localized areas of necrosis. Symptoms may include decreased motor control of facial and extremity musculature, clumsiness, diffuse sensory disturbances, and dysarthria.

Cerebral Vascular Accident— Popular Intervention Concepts

Bobath Technique Neuro-developmental Treatment (NDT)

The goal of these techniques is to normalize muscle tone, inhibit abnormal motor patterns, and facilitate normal motion.

The techniques include moving the patient through a variety of movement patterns that activate neurological processes associated with or requisite for normal motion.

Brunnstrom Technique

The Brunnstrom approach is characterized by the identification of definitive stages of motor recovery and stereotypical movement patterns known as synergies.

The goal of treatment is to facilitate movement within the recovery stage and to gradually facilitate transition to the next recovery stage.

It is primarily a movement facilitative technique. The technique includes the facilitation of movement using associated reactions, reflexive motion, and the gradual combination of movement components of divergent synergies.

Rood Technique

This technique is characterized by the use of sensory stimulation such as brushing, icing, and vibration to facilitate or inhibit muscle contraction or tone.

Complex Regional Pain Syndrome/ Reflex Sympathetic Dystrophy

Classification Complex Regional Pain Syndrome (CRPS), formerly called Reflex Sympathetic Dystrophy (RSD), is a posttraumatic neuropathic condition. CRPS is usually associated with pain of one or more limbs. CRPS may be seen post Colles and other fractures, sprains, peripheral nerve injuries, falls, cardiovascular accident, myocardial infarction, or cervical arthritis. It may begin in one part of an extremity and progress proximally.

Manifestations **Type I** CRPS occurs when nerve injury cannot be immediately identified. **Type II** CRPS, also known as causalgia, occurs when a distinctive major nerve injury has occurred.

Initial CRPS symptoms include pain, warmth, erythema, rapid nail growth, and edema in the hand. These symptoms may progress to burning and hyperesthesia that increase with the onset of cold weather.

Other symptoms of CRPS may also include weakness, fatigue, skin rash, shiny skin, vasomotor instability, increased bone resorption, frequent infections, and migraine headaches. Symptoms can last from 6 months to longer than a year; they can subside and recur later.

Medical Management Diagnosis of CRPS is made through history and physical examination. Medical management of CRPS consists of medications, relaxation training, hypnosis, and guarded imagery.

Opioids, NSAIDS, tricyclic antidepressants, antiepileptic, and muscle relaxants are used in the treatment of CRPS. It is also treated with sympathetic nerve blocks and in rare instances implanting of a dorsal column stimulator.   *continues*

Complex Regional Pain Syndrome/ Reflex Sympathetic Dystrophy, cont.

Psychological support and physical therapy may be prescribed. As a last resort, physicians may inject Ziconotide, a nonopioid anesthetic, through a catheter into the patient's spinal fluid. The best treatment is prevention by keeping the extremity moving, minimizing edema, and monitoring vascularity.

Physical Therapy Goals

Patients with CRPS are seen on an outpatient basis. Initial goals involve pain and edema control along with mobilizing the extremity. Other goals include desensitizing the involved area and patient education stressing the importance of increasing activity and movement.

Effective PT Interventions

Initial goals of pain and edema reduction may be achieved through the use of modalities including ultrasound, TENS, or ice. Compression stockings, intermittent compression modalities, and massage can be effective in decreasing edema.

Biofeedback may be used to increase relaxation thereby changing blood flow. Treatment for CRPS should also include improving range of motion and strength within the pain-free range.

In addition to isotonic and isometric exercise, closed chain activities should be used to improve strength of the entire extremity. Aquatic therapy has been shown to be effective. Desensitization techniques such as tapping, gentle brushing, rubbing, or fluidotherapy may be effective in decreasing hypersensitivity.

Precautions

Stretching should not be performed when the patient is in pain.

Cystic Fibrosis

Classification	Cystic fibrosis (CF) is a genetic disease affecting approximately 30,000 children and adults in the United States. It is characterized by the production of abnormally thick, sticky mucus. This mucus clogs the lungs leading to infections and airway blockages. The thick mucus also obstructs pancreatic and bile ducts leading to organ damage and severe digestive impairments.
Manifestations	A major diagnostic manifestation of this disease is high sodium and chloride concentrations in the sweat. The overproduction of thick mucus leads to life-threatening pulmonary, gastrointestinal, cardiac, hepatic, and pancreatic complications. The median life span for an individual with CF is just over 30 years.
Medical Management	Medical management includes antibiotics, supplemental digestive enzymes, and vitamins. NSAIDS are used to manage inflammation, especially of lung tissue.
Physical Therapy Goals	The major physical therapy goal is the clearance of mucus and fluids from the lung fields.
Effective PT Interventions	Postural drainage and chest physical therapy are effective physical therapy interventions. These interventions may be performed two to three times per day.
	Auscultation must be carefully performed to direct postural drainage to affected lung fields.
	Patient, caregiver, and parental education and instruction in postural drainage and pulmonary hygiene techniques are also important.
Precautions	Postural drainage should not be performed just before or immediately after meals.

continues

Guillain-Barre Syndrome

Classification

Guillain-Barre Syndrome (GBS) is an acute inflammatory demyelinating polyradiculopathy. GBS is thought to be autoimmune in origin.

Manifestations

GBS is characterized by progressive distal to proximal muscle weakness, which may progress to the muscles of respiration leading to respirator dependence.

There is a spontaneous cessation of symptoms followed by gradual recovery; often residual distal lower extremity weakness persists.

Medical Management

Plasmapheresis—the removal, filtering, and then replacement of plasma—is an effective procedure. This procedure helps to dilute or filter circulating antibodies. High-dose IV immunoglobulin administration is also effective.

Comprehensive rehabilitation services are prescribed during recovery.

Physical Therapy Goals

Initial goals include preservation of ROM through positioning and splinting. Maintenance of pulmonary status is accomplished with postural drainage, percussion, and vibration.

Rehabilitation goals include the restoration of normal ROM, strength, and functional abilities.

Effective PT Interventions

Given the proximal to distal return of muscle function, closed chain lower extremity activities are helpful in early rehabilitation.

Isokinetic and isotonic exercises for large muscle groups are effective. Given multiple muscle group involvement, aquatic therapy (if available) is of great benefit.

Use of lower extremity orthotics may be indicated to enhance safety and manage residual weakness.

Guillain-Barre Syndrome, cont.

Use of assistive gait devices may be indicated during recovery.

Precautions   Avoid overworking and excessive fatigue.

Low Back Pain

Classification   Low back pain (LBP) is the number one cause of short-term disability in the United States. Typically low back pain encompasses discomfort in the lower thoracic, lumbar, and sacral regions. Low back pain can be acute or chronic.

A popular school of thought is that most low back pain can be traced to mechanical and postural anomalies precipitated by assuming poor sitting postures, improper lifting techniques, and employing anatomically inappropriate movement patterns. These factors may lead to injury of bony and soft tissue structures, maladaptive shortening of soft tissue, and adverse forces at the intervertebral disk.

Manifestations   Low back pain is characterized by a varying degree of discomfort. Discomfort may be characterized as nuisance pain with little disability or severe pain with significant disability. Nerve root irritation, radiating pain, neurogenic muscle weakness, and sensory changes may be associated with the discomfort.

Some clinicians subdivide low back pain into three distinct syndromes: postural syndrome, dysfunction syndrome, and derangement syndrome. Though the syndromes are individually defined, they are not mutually exclusive and the presence of one syndrome may precipitate another.

continues

Low Back Pain, cont.

Postural Syndrome: This syndrome occurs when the lumbar spine is held in a relatively static position. Soft tissues surrounding the bony structures are placed under prolonged stress. In the postural syndrome, the patient only complains of symptoms when the stressful posture is assumed.

Dysfunction Syndrome: This syndrome occurs as a result of maladaptive shortening of spinal soft tissue precipitating a loss of mobility. Soft tissues are prematurely elongated before full range of motion is achieved. The premature stretching of these tissues causes pain.

Derangement Syndrome: This syndrome occurs as a result of an alteration to the normal resting position of two adjacent vertebrae secondary to a change in the position of the interspersed nucleus pulposis. Changes in pulposis position may lead to a varying degree of spinal cord, nerve root, or vascular compression.

Medical Management

Low back pain is typically managed with a combination of pain medications, NSAIDS, rest from normal functions, and physical therapy. Diagnosis may be made based upon physical examination and medical imaging such as CT and MRI scans, myelograms, and traditional X-rays.

In severe cases, surgical management may be indicated. Surgical procedures such as laminectomy and discectomy are performed to relieve nerve root compression.

In chronic low back pain, management often involves a team approach including psychological support, medical management, physical rehabilitation intervention, vocational counseling, dietary management, and other professional input.

Low Back Pain, cont.

Physical Therapy Goals

Initial physical therapy goals address pain management. As pain is managed, goals related to the restoration of range of motion, strength, and normal posture are emphasized. Treatment of the root cause of the symptoms is considered.

Low back pain is most often associated with postural or mechanical factors. Even the nature of acute low back pain is relatively long term. Therefore, it is crucial that patient education goals be established.

Physical therapy treatment includes teaching the patient how to recognize the precipitating factors and how to best manage their pain. This often includes alteration in posture, workplace modifications, alteration in activities of daily living, and effective participation in home exercise. Ideally, the patient should become increasingly more reliant upon self-treatment strategies for the management of their pain rather than formal physical therapy services.

Effective PT Interventions

Modalities can be effective in treating low back pain. Modalities most often used include electrical stimulation, moist heat, and ultrasound.

TENS should be provided in an ambulatory fashion; that is, the patient should be allowed to perform functional activities while receiving the treatment.

Therapeutic exercises should be prescribed according to the patient's level of disability, root cause of symptoms, and amount of pain.

Rather than simply performing a group of generic low back exercises, exercises should be carefully selected. Specific sets of exercises are associated

continues

Low Back Pain, cont.

with the treatment of postural, dysfunction, and derangement syndromes. These exercises should be selectively prescribed based upon the patient's particular diagnosis. The chapter on therapeutic exercise in this text reviews exercises that are effective in managing low back pain.

Precautions   Special emphasis must be placed on the correct performance of therapeutic exercise. Lumbar flexion with rotation should be avoided and appropriate body mechanics stressed.

Multiple Sclerosis

Classification   Multiple sclerosis (MS) is progressive neurological disease. MS involves demyelination of neurons of the brain, spinal cord, and cranial nerves. The demyelination affects sensory, motor, and autonomic fibers. It affects women at twice the rate of men with initial onset most commonly occurring between the ages of 20 and 40. Etiology is unknown, although studies suggest genetic, immunologic, and environmental factors.

Manifestations   Clinical manifestations of MS vary greatly. In some cases visual problems may include diplopia (blurred vision), gaze palsies, scotoma (a spot in the visual field), nystagmus (involuntary rhythmic tremor of the eye), decreased color vision, visual field defects, and reduced clarity of vision.

Sensory deficits include paresthesias (tingling, pricking) or hypoesthesia (decreased sensitivity). Depression and cognitive changes may occur. Some patients experience memory loss, impaired judgment, dysarthria (poor articulation), incontinence, exaggerated tendon reflexes, pain, and fatigue.

Multiple Sclerosis, cont.

Some patients complain of persistent tiredness and/or fatigue after exercise. Motor problems include spasticity, stiffness, slowness, weakness, clonus, spontaneous spasms, decreased balance and coordination.

MS is categorized into four general categories:

1. Relapse and Remitting. With each relapse (or exacerbation), new symptoms occur or previous symptoms get worse. Each relapse may last a number of days to a number of months with partial to total recovery each time. This accounts for 25% of the population.

2. Benign. The patient experiences one or two attacks with no residual disability. This accounts for 20% of the population.

3. Secondary Progressive. Initially, the patient will have periods of relapse and remittance, then develop a progressive disability with later superimposed relapses. This accounts for 40% of the population.

4. Primary Progressive. With this type, there is a slow onset, then sudden worsening of symptoms. This accounts for 15% of the population.

Medical Management

There is no cure for MS. However, many drugs have been found to decrease symptoms and increase the time between relapses. During the acute stage of a relapse, patients are usually treated with corticosteroids (prednisone, methylprednisone, or dexamethasone).

Long-term drug treatments include the use of interferon beta 1a or 1b (i.e., avonex, betaseron) or copaxone. Other drugs are used to treat specific
continues

Multiple Sclerosis, cont.

symptoms. Tegretol, Neurontin, and Dilantin are used to treat acute pain while Elavil and Wellbutrin are used in treating more chronic pain.

Leg spasms and back pain are treated with NSAIDS, Lioresal, Zanaflex, Valium, or Dantrolene. New drug treatments are currently being developed and studied.

Physical Therapy Goals

PT management of MS occurs in inpatient and outpatient settings dependent on the severity of symptoms. In an acute care setting, initial goals focus on function such as bed mobility, transfers and ambulation, and/or wheelchair mobility depending on the patient's individual current and past functional status.

Inpatient rehabilitation goals continue to focus on function as well as improving strength, balance, and coordination.

Outpatient goals are dependent on the needs of the patient. Functional goals are aimed at making the patient as independent as possible in bed mobility, transfers, ambulation and gait, and wheelchair mobility.

Goals may also address strength, pain management, balance and coordination, normalization of tone, and endurance training. To make goals more measurable, impairment and disability scales may be used.

Effective PT Interventions

PT intervention will depend on the patient's current and past functional status. Initial treatment may focus on functional training as well as training patient in the use of assistive devices and aids.

Multiple Sclerosis, cont.

Care should be given to maintain and/or improve ROM. Strengthening exercises begin with open chain exercises and progress to close chain activities depending on the patient's functional status. Strengthening should be performed submaximally to help avoid fatigue.

Isotonic exercise using light weights and elastic resistives, as well as aerobic activities including walking, cycling, and swimming, may be effective in maintaining function.

Endurance training, as well as sitting-and-standing balance and coordination activities should be emphasized. Home exercise programs and patient education should emphasize stretching and strengthening activities as well as the importance of routine exercise during periods of relapse and remittance. Patients need to learn to recognize their own signs of fatigue and take periods of rest.

Neurological symptoms such as changes in muscle tone are addressed through a variety of neurodevelopmental techniques including principles put forth by Bobath, Rood, Brunnstrom, etc.

Precautions　　Patients should avoid exercising for long periods of time. Hot baths, increased body temperatures, and hot weather can cause fatigue and worsen symptoms.

The clinician must consider that the apparent muscle weakness is a result of atrophy of muscle fibers still under voluntary control and the impairment of central influence.

continues

Multiple Sclerosis, cont.

The clinician must not lose sight of the central nervous system origin of the disease. Strengthening activities do not result in increased control of musculature directly affected by the disease. However, strengthening of muscles under volitional control may improve function.

Osteoarthritis

Classification

Osteoarthritis (OA) is otherwise known as degenerative joint disease (DJD). OA is a slow, progressive degenerative disease. Wear and tear is thought to play a role in the emergence of this disease. OA affects articular cartilage of synovial joints. As the disease progresses, patients may experience bony remodeling, formation of spurs, and synovial and capsular thickening.

These changes in synovial joints may lead to contractures, loss of ROM, pain, and instability. The weight-bearing joints are most often affected. There is no known cause for primary arthritis although links have been made to aging and genetic predisposition.

Secondary OA is also known as traumatic arthritis. The causes of secondary arthritis include trauma, fractures, infection, and osteonecrosis. Secondary OA may result from sport activities, obesity, or repetitive kneeling or squatting activities.

Manifestations

Symptoms typically progress slowly. Patients may complain of pain, stiffness, loss of flexibility, swelling, crepitus, tenderness upon palpation, limited ROM, and decreased function.

Patients may have stiffness after periods of rest and pain with activity, especially weight-bearing

Osteoarthritis, cont.

	activities. As the disease progresses, patients may develop deformities secondary to degenerative changes of accessory joint structures. As activity levels decrease, patients may experience muscle weakness.
Medical Management	Medical diagnosis is made by physical examination and radiological tests. Physicians may prescribe medication, assistive devices, and physical and occupational therapy. NSAIDS are used to decrease inflammation and relieve pain. In severe cases where patients have developed deformities, contractures, destruction of articular cartilage, and decreased function joint replacement may be indicated.
Physical Therapy Goals	Patients with OA who have not had surgery are usually seen in an outpatient setting. The goals of therapy depend on the patients' level of function and progression of the disease. Goals may include decreasing pain, preventing or minimizing contractures, and improving function.
	Goals to enhance ROM, strength, endurance, joint preservation, and patient education are also pursued.
Effective PT Interventions	Modalities and exercise are used to control pain. Thermal and electrical stimulation modalities are used. Exercise may include active ROM and resistive exercise depending on the patients' strength and pain.
	To alleviate stress of the joint and improve function, physical therapy may include transfer, ambulation, and balance training. Patient education involves teaching home exercise programs and instruction in the use of assistive devices.

continues

Patients with OA of the hip usually require exercise for hip abduction and extension in particular. Patients with OA of the knee usually require exercise for quadriceps and hamstrings. Patient may also need education in care and use of orthotic and assistive devices.

Precautions   If excessive pain occurs during or after resistive exercise, resistance should be reduced.

Parkinson's Disease

Classification   Parkinson's disease is a chronic progressive neuromuscular disorder. Parkinson's disease is the result of a loss of or impairment of cells in the substantia nigra of the brain. This leads to a decreased production of the neurotransmitter dopamine, which causes a decreased ability to direct or control movement. The cause of Parkinson's disease is unknown. Links to genetic and environmental causes are being researched. Onset typically occurs after the age of 50, although 10% of incidences occur under the age of 40.

Manifestations   The most common clinical manifestations include rigidity and resting tremor. Initially, symptoms may occur in one extremity before progressing to other extremities and the trunk. As the disease progresses, patients may develop balance deficits and gait deviations.

A shuffling gait, characterized by decreased step length, hip flexion, and ankle dorsiflexion are often seen in people with Parkinson's disease. Other manifestations include bradykinesia (slow movement), dyskinesia, poor posture, decreased facial expressions, muffled speech, and depression.

Parkinson's Disease, cont.

Most patients experience weakness and fatigue as the disease continues to progress. In 50% of cases, the disease progresses to dementia and intellectual changes. However, some of these changes may be facilitated by side effects associated with pharmaceutical management of the disease. Progression of this disease may be fast or slow.

Medical Management

There is no cure for Parkinson's disease. Diagnosis is made through physical examination. Medications do not stop the progression of the disease but help to treat the symptoms.

Levodopa (sinamet) is used to increase mobility. Other medications include anticholinergic drugs, comatin (eldepryl), parlodel, pernox, mirapex, cogentin, symmetril, artane, and bromocriptine.

Surgery may be indicated in extreme cases. One surgery is a pallidotomy in which an electric probe is inserted into the brain to destroy the global pallidus. This helps to control dyskinesia. A thalamotomy destroys cells in thalamus and helps control arm/hand tremors. A new procedure involves deep brain stimulation. Electrodes are implanted in the brain and connected to an external pulse generator. This procedure has been shown to decrease tremors.

Physical Therapy Goals

Patients with Parkinson's disease may be seen in inpatient (rehabilitation facilities or nursing homes), outpatient, or home care settings. In acute care, patients may be seen with a secondary diagnosis of Parkinson's disease.

continues

Parkinson's Disease, cont.

PT goals focus on increasing mobility and improving function. Specific goals are dependent on how far the disease has progressed. At initial stages, goals may focus on improving and maintaining posture, maintaining mobility, and increasing strength. Other goals may include improvement and maintenance of gait, balance, and general ADL.

Effective PT Interventions

In early stages of the disease, treatment may focus on improving posture and patient education. Treatment involves neck and trunk control exercises to decrease forward head and kyphosis. Reaching activities may emphasize trunk rotation and reinforce improved posture. Cones may be used for reaching exercises.

Gait training includes improving step length, increasing base of support, and improving arm swing. Obstacle courses may emphasize increase step length and hip flexion. Patients can step over objects such as canes or cones. Variable spacing of obstacles may enforce increased step length. Patients should be closely guarded during all ambulation activities.

Due to rigidity and dyskinesia symptoms, patients may have decreased range of motion and weakness. Stretching and strengthening programs may be needed. Home exercise programs include stretching and strengthening exercise and posture education.

Home exercise programs are dependent on how far the disease has progressed. Patients may require assistance with their home exercise program and therefore family members and caregivers should be involved in the education process.

Precautions

Given the loss of movement control and the presence of rigidity, safety precautions related to gait and ADL must always be emphasized.

Piriformis Syndrome

Classification
Piriformis syndrome is a neuromuscular disorder resulting in irritation or compression of the sciatic nerve due to spasm or contracture of the piriformis muscle. Piriformis syndrome has been found to be more prevalent in women and has become more commonly seen in runners and walkers.

A number of etiologies have been proposed including hyperlordosis, hypertrophy of the piriformis muscle, trauma, hip flexion contracture, cerebral palsy, total hip arthroplasty, ischial bursitis, excessive activity, inflammation or spasm of the piriformis muscle, and anatomical abnormalities.

Manifestations
The most common clinical manifestation is pain in the buttocks and posterior thigh. Other manifestations may include tingling and numbness down the sciatic nerve and pain radiating to the foot. However, it should be noted that piriformis syndrome does not cause true sciatica.

Medical Management
Piriformis syndrome is diagnosed through physical examination. Nonsteroidal anti-inflammatory drugs such as ibuprofen or naproxen are used to assist in decreasing inflammation. In severe cases, injections of a local anesthetic and corticosteroid may be used to decrease spasm and alleviate sciatic pain. In rare cases, a muscle weakening agent such as botulinum toxin may be injected into the area.

Physical Therapy Goals
PT management of piriformis syndrome is usually on an outpatient basis. Initial findings other than complaints of pain may include tight piriformis, limited hip internal rotation and abduction, weak hip abduction, lower lumbar spine dysfunction, sacroiliac hypomobility, decreased stride length, limb length shortening, and hip external rotation with ambulation.

continues

Piriformis Syndrome, cont.

Initial goals are to manage pain as well as decreasing muscle spasms and contractures. As pain decreases, the goals will focus on increasing flexibility and strength, ambulation training (addressing gait deviations), and patient education.

Effective PT Interventions

In the early stage of treatment, emphasis is on pain management including the use of modalities and stretching. Modalities often used include electrical stimulation specifically TENS and interferential current stimulations to block pain and decrease spasm and ice.

Passive and self stretching of the piriformis, hamstrings, hip extensors, and hip rotators are important. Muscle spasm of the piriformis is often palpable and deep massage is performed to address the spasm.

Strengthening of muscles and addressing gait deviations is emphasized as the patient progresses. Home exercise program includes self stretches for the piriformis and hamstrings.

Patient education regarding prevention and proper body mechanics is also crucial. While being treated for piriformis syndrome, patients should avoid bicycling, running, and similar activities.

Precautions

Because emphasis is placed on self-management, patients must be carefully instructed in passive self-stretching ensuring the avoidance of ballistic-type stretching.

Rheumatoid Arthritis

Classification

Rheumatoid arthritis (RA) is a chronic systemic disease. RA is an inflammatory disease with an unknown etiology. Joints commonly affected are the cervical spine, wrist, knees, and joints of the

Rheumatoid Arthritis, cont.

fingers, hands, and feet. Other systems that may be affected by the disease include the cardiovascular, pulmonary, gastrointestinal, ocular, and skeletal.

Manifestations

Symptoms of RA vary from mild to severe. It may begin suddenly and progress slowly. Patients also experience periods of exacerbations and remissions.

Patients may experience acute inflammatory periods followed by subacute and chronic periods.

Stage I involves swelling of the synovial lining which leads to pain, warmth, stiffness, redness, and swelling around the joint. **Stage II** involves a rapid division and growth of cells leading to synovial thickening. **Stage III** occurs when inflamed cells release enzymes that digest bone and cartilage. This may lead to changes in the shape of the joints and changes in joint alignment. As a result, patient may experience more pain and loss of mobility.

Other patient complaints may include fatigue, weakness, edema, and stiffness. Involvement is usually symmetrical. Ulnar deviation, swan-neck, and boutoniere deformities are seen in patients with RA.

Medical Management

Diagnosis of RA is made through history, physical examination, and laboratory tests.

Medical management of RA includes medication and referrals to physical and occupational therapy. Studies have shown aggressive drug treatment during initial symptoms can limit future joint damage. Medications include multiple antirheumatic drugs along with prednisone or infiximab (Remicade).

When RA leads to degeneration of the joints, surgeries such as total joint replacements may be indicated.

continues

Rheumatoid Arthritis, cont.

Synovectomy at the wrist/hand complex may be performed to treat pain and improve function.

Physical Therapy Goals

Physical therapy goals vary depending on the stage of the disease process.

During periods of exacerbation, initial goals include pain reduction, maintaining mobility, minimizing stiffness, patient education, conserving of energy, and introducing functional modifications. When applicable, patient goals may also include those pertaining to transfer and ambulation training.

As the inflammatory response dissipates, goals focus on strengthening, gentle stretching, increasing physical activity, endurance training, and home exercise programs. Limiting deformity and maximizing function are important goals.

Effective PT Interventions

Pain reduction includes the use of modalities, gentle massage, splinting, and relaxation techniques.

Active ROM exercises are used to maintain motion and minimize stiffness.

Patients are encouraged to continue activities of daily living to further minimize stiffness. Patients need to be taught to conserve energy and monitor fatigue.

Patients are educated to identify signs of fatigue and inflammation and limit stresses on the body during times of exacerbation.

The use of assistive devices that preserve joint alignment and reduce weight-bearing forces are effective in reducing pain and maximizing function.

Regular guarded community activity such as swimming, low-impact aerobics, and light cycling help maintain function between exacerbations.

Rheumatoid Arthritis, cont.

When possible, patients should be referred to community organizations that facilitate these types of activities.

During the subacute and chronic stages, gentle stretching exercises may be performed to prevent or minimize contractures.

Postsurgical patients are treated based upon a prescribed protocol and the nature of the surgery. Postsurgical physical therapy typically includes modalities for inflammation management, gentle stretching, strengthening activities, gait and transfer activities.

Precautions   Stretching should be avoided during acute inflammatory stages. Vigorous stretching is always contraindicated. Fatigue during therapeutic exercise should be avoided. Deep soft tissue and manipulation techniques are contraindicated.

Rotator Cuff Injury

Classification   Rotator cuff injury is characterized by damage to one or more of the rotator cuff tendons (supraspinatus, infraspinatus, teres minor, subcapularis). The pathology is typically caused by repetitive use or trauma.

Manifestations   Typical clinical manifestations include pain with shoulder motion, especially overhead motion, loss of range of motion, and decreased muscle strength.

Medical Management   Diagnosis can be made with a thorough physical examination. Effective medical imaging includes MRI, arthrogram, and sonography.

continues

Rotator Cuff Injury, cont.

Most cuff injuries are treated conservatively with NSAIDS and/or corticosteroid injections. Surgical management includes physical repair of the tendon(s) by arthroscopic or open surgery.

Physical Therapy Goals

Physical therapy goals include the restoration of shoulder strength and ROM and the maintenance of strength and ROM of the noninvolved joints.

Effective PT Interventions

Physical therapy intervention is often protocol based. Popular protocols outline therapeutic interventions for 12–18 weeks.

Generally, protocols are not standardized. Protocols are based on the extensiveness of the repair and the conservatism and experience of the surgeon. All protocols are characterized by gradual progression of ROM and strengthening activities.

Precautions

Precautions may change depending upon postoperative phase. For instance, for the first 3 to 4 weeks, only pendulum exercises may be indicated. The PTA should obtain a written copy of the protocol from the physical therapist and follow it carefully.

Scoliosis

Classification

Scoliosis is an abnormal lateral curvature of the spine. In most cases of scoliosis, the cause is unknown. Other causes of scoliosis are secondary to spinal disease, bony abnormality, or neurological disorders. Onset may occur at birth, juvenile age (4–10 years old), or adolescence.

Manifestations

The curvature may be toward the right or the left. Most commonly observed curves involve a right thoracic, left lumbar curve (otherwise called an S-curve) or a left thoracolumbar curve (otherwise called a C-curve).

Scoliosis, cont.

Scoliosis may be termed structural or nonstructural (functional). Functional (or postural) scoliosis is reversible. Typically, the curve disappears or decreases when the patient flexes forward or is supine. Functional scoliosis may develop secondary to leg length discrepancies, postural problems, or spasms of the spinal column muscles.

Structural or irreversible scoliosis cannot be reduced or eliminated with change in position. Along with the lateral curvature, patients with structural curves often display a rotation of the vertebrae.

Curvatures result in asymmetrical shoulder levels and/or uneven pelvic levels. Depending on the severity, scoliosis may produce pulmonary problems, muscle imbalance, decreased flexibility, overstretched muscles, back pain, degenerative spinal arthritis, disk disease, vertebral subluxation, or sciatica.

Medical Management

Scoliosis is diagnosed through physical examination and radiological tests. Patients with structural scoliosis may be managed through conservative or nonconservative management.

Conservative management involves spinal bracing otherwise known as a thoracic-lumbosacral orthosis (TLSO). The TLSO is worn 23 hours a day for a period of time ranging from months to years. It should be noted that bracing does not correct the deformity but slows progression of the curvature.

Functional electrical stimulation is a controversial conservative treatment. Electrodes are placed on the back on the convex side of the curve at night while the patient is sleeping.

continues

Scoliosis, cont.

Nonconservative management involves spinal surgery. Surgery is done on patients with severe curvatures. The surgery involves spinal fusion and the use of rods and chains to stabilize the spinal column. After surgery, surgeons may cast or brace the patient for a period of time during the healing process.

Physical Therapy Goals

Physical therapy goals are dependent on medical management. In conservative management, patients may be seen on an outpatient basis. The goal of physical therapy is to maintain posture and function.

Effective PT Interventions

Physical therapy for patients who are conservatively managed involves patient education and maintenance of posture. Treatment involves postural awareness, flexibility maintenance, and strengthening of spinal muscles.

Exercises include strengthening of the trunk extensors, abdominals, and gluteal muscles, and stretching the trunk extensors and iliopsoas muscles. Emphasis is placed on self management.

Patients that are treated surgically are seen in the hospital for bed mobility and functional training as well as exercise. Patients are instructed in log rolling and transfer and ambulation training if needed.

Exercises include deep breathing exercises, AROM and muscle setting (i.e., quad sets) to maintain strength and ankle pumps for circulation.

Surgical patients are seen in outpatient facilities following discharge from the hospital. Treatment includes flexibility and strengthening exercises of the lower extremities as well as trunk

Scoliosis, cont.

strengthening. Patients in casts or wearing braces should be instructed in proper skin care.

Precautions   Postsurgical precautions include avoiding excessive bending, trunk rotation, and trunk hyperextension. Patients may have lifting restrictions.

Thoracic Outlet Syndrome

Classification   Thoracic Outlet Syndrome (TOS) incorporates a number of diagnoses involving upper extremity neurological and vascular symptoms of the thoracic outlet. The thoracic outlet is an anatomical space where vascular structures and nerves of the brachial plexus enter the arm between the clavicle and first rib. Entrapment may involve nerves and/or arteries. Causes of TOS may include compressive neuropathy, faulty posture, trauma to the shoulder girdle, and entrapment.

Manifestations   Symptoms of TOS vary from patient to patient depending on whether there is nerve or vascular involvement. Patients with neurological involvement complain of paresthesias in the arm especially when they are sleeping and when the arm is elevated above 90°.

Other symptoms may include numbness, weakness, discoloration, swelling, ulceration, gangrene, and in some cases, Raynaud's phenomenon. Complaints of neck, shoulder, or radiating pain to the hand are common. Complaints also include difficulty sleeping and difficulty carrying objects, especially on the shoulder.

Medical Management   Management may be nonoperative or operative. Diagnosis involves physical examination. Radiological and electrophysiological tests may be performed for differential diagnosis.   *continues*

Thoracic Outlet Syndrome, cont.

Initial nonoperative treatment usually consists of physical therapy. In extreme cases where conservative treatment fails, surgery may be indicated.

Surgical procedures for TOS are scalenectomy, clavicle resection, pectoralis major release, and first rib resection.

Physical Therapy Goals

Patients with TOS are usually seen in the outpatient setting. Goals are dependent on patient symptoms and etiology. Initially the goal is to increase mobility in the thoracic outlet. This may be accomplished through improving posture and strengthening postural muscles. Other goals include increasing ROM, mobilizing nerve tissue, and improving respiratory function.

Effective PT Interventions

Initial treatment focuses on patient education. Postural exercises and the importance of decreasing stress on the thoracic outlet are emphasized.

Early stages of treatment involve pain management and inflammation. Other treatments include stretching and strengthening.

Scalenes, pectoralis minor and major, anterior portion of the intercostals, and short suboccipital muscles typically require stretching.

Common muscles needing strengthening include scapular adductors and upward rotators, trapezius, levator scapulae, rhomboids, shoulder medial rotators, short anterior cervical muscles, and thoracic extensors.

Breathing exercises are taught when respiratory patterns are impaired. Breathing exercises include deep breathing and diaphragmatic breathing exercises.

Thoracic Outlet Syndrome, cont.

Precautions   Overhead exercises and activities that elicit symptoms and forceful stretching that mobilizes the first rib should be avoided.

Total Hip Replacement

Classification   Total hip replacement (THR) is most often performed in the management of severe osteoarthritis (OA). The procedure is indicated for patients with severe limitations in movement and function, instability of the hip, deformity, and pain. Other indications for THR not associated with osteoarthritis include rheumatoid arthritis, bone cancer, avascular necrosis, and hip fracture.

Surgical/Medical Management   A THR consists of the replacement of the proximal femur and the insertion of an acetabular cup. Implants are typically made of metal, but allografts are also used.

To secure the artificial joint components, a special surgical cement may be used to fill the gap between the prosthesis and remaining natural bone. Noncemented prostheses may be used for younger, more active patients. These prostheses are coated with a textured metal or a specialized substance that allows bone to grow into the prostheses and secure it.

There are a number of surgical approaches including the posterolateral, lateral, and anterolateral. Each of these approaches has advantages and disadvantages as well as associated rehabilitation precautions.

Postoperatively, patients will return to their room with intravenous antibiotics and pain medications. The surgical incision is held together with staples that are later removed. Patients will also have an abduction wedge placed between the lower

continues

Total Hip Replacement, cont.

	extremities to keep the hip abducted while the patient is in bed. Weight-bearing status is dependent on the physician's orders and whether the hip is cemented.
Physical Therapy Goals	Initial postoperative physical therapy goals concentrate on transfer, bed mobility, and ambulation training. Increasing hip ROM, minimizing muscle atrophy, and patient education is also important. As patients progress, goals focus on strengthening, endurance training, and minimizing gait deviations.
Effective PT Interventions	Initially, patients will be seen 1 or 2 days after surgery in an acute care setting. Treatment involves transfer and ambulation training. Weight-bearing status needs to be confirmed by the doctors' orders and/or the physical therapy treatment plan.
	Walkers are usually used to begin ambulation. Patients are often progressed to loftstrand crutches or a cane. Initial activities include muscle setting AROM and AAROM exercises. Gluteal, quadriceps, and hamstring setting exercises are performed. Resistive exercises are performed on the unaffected side.
	Examples of AROM and AAROM include heel slides, hip abduction in the spine, short arc quadriceps, knee flexion and extension, and ankle pumps. Deep breathing exercises are also important. In addition, patients need to be taught total hip precautions and home exercise programs.
	Once released from acute care, patients may be discharged to inpatient rehabilitation, skilled nursing facilities, or home depending on their functional abilities. As patients progress, treatment advances to strengthening, balance, and endurance training exercises.

Total Hip Replacement, cont.

Cold therapy and electrical stimulation may be used to decrease pain and edema. Once independent in ambulation and cleared for full weight bearing, patient may begin closed chain exercises and slow, high-seat stationary cycling. However, total hip precautions must be maintained at all times.

Precautions   **Posterolateral approach**: Avoid hip flexion greater than 80° to 90°, adduction past neutral, and internal rotation past neutral.

Anterolateral and lateral approach: Avoid hip flexion greater than 80° to 90° and adduction past neutral. Avoid extension past neutral and external rotation past neutral. In addition, avoid combining hip flexion, abduction, and external rotation.

ADL precautions: Regardless of surgical approach, patients should:

- Not sit on low, soft seats
- Not cross their legs
- Not bend over or flex the trunk forward
- Use a commode or raised toilet seat
- Avoid sleeping in sidelying
- Use a shower or tub chair
- Transfer in and out of bed leading with the affected limb
- Avoid pivoting on the affected lower extremity

These precautions decrease the risk of hip dislocation.

Total Knee Replacement

Classification   Total knee replacements (TKRs) may be indicated for patients with marked limitations in motion, joint instability, destruction of articular cartilage, marked deformity, pain, and limitations in function.

continues

Total Knee Replacement, cont.

Surgical/Medical Management   TKRs involve a replacement of the distal femur and proximal tibia and occasional resurfacing of the patella with metal implants.

To secure the artificial joint components, a special surgical cement may be used to fill the gap between the prosthesis and remaining natural bone. Noncemented prostheses may be used for younger, more active patients. These prostheses are coated with a textured metal or a specialized substance that allows bone to grow into the prostheses and secure it.

There are a number of surgical approaches including the anterior, subvastus, and lateral. Incisions are held together with staples or sutures.

Postoperatively, the surgical site is dressed with a compression bandage and a knee immobilizer may be applied. Pain medication and antibiotics may also be prescribed.

Physical Therapy Goals   Initial postoperative physical therapy goals concentrate on transfer and ambulation training. Increasing knee ROM, minimizing muscle atrophy, and patient education is also important.

Early knee ROM is essential. If not achieved early in the healing process, lack of motion and function may be permanent. Patients need at least 90° of flexion for functional activities including normal sitting, transferring in and out of cars, or negotiating stairs. Without full knee extension, patients will display gait deviations. As the patient progresses, goals focus on strengthening, endurance training, and minimizing gait deviations.

Total Knee Replacement, cont.

Effective PT Interventions

Initially, patients will be seen 1 or 2 days after surgery in an acute care setting. Treatment involves transfer and ambulation training. Weight-bearing status needs to be confirmed by the doctors' orders and/or the physical therapy treatment plan.

Walkers are usually used to begin ambulation. Depending on the physician's orders, patient may not need to wear knee immobilizer when ambulating. However, knee immobilizers are used to maintain terminal knee extension and many patients sleep with the immobilizer applied.

Patients are often progressed to loftstrand crutches or a cane. Initial activities include muscle setting, and AROM and AAROM exercises. Gluteal, quadriceps, and hamstring setting exercises are performed.

Continuous passive motion (CPM) machines are sometimes used for knee flexion and extension ROM. Resistive exercises are performed on the unaffected side.

Examples of AROM and AAROM to affected side include heel slides, short arc quadriceps, straight-leg raises, and ankle pumps. Deep breathing exercises are also important. In addition, patients need to be taught a home exercise program.

Once released from acute care, patients may be discharged to inpatient rehabilitation, skilled nursing facilities, or home depending on their functional abilities. As patients progress, treatment advances to strengthening, balance, and endurance training exercises. Cold therapy and electrical stimulation may be used to decrease pain and edema.

Once independent in ambulation and cleared for full weight bearing, patient may begin closed chain exercises, and stationary cycling.

continues

Total Knee Replacement, cont.

Precautions	Avoid using a pillow under the knee postoperatively because it may cause a knee flexion contraction. Carefully monitor the integrity of the incision during knee flexion.

Trochanteric Bursitis

Classification	Trochanteric bursitis is caused by acute or repetitive trauma to the bursa that lies just superficial to the greater trochanter. Repetitive trauma is often attributed to friction irritation from the illiotibial band. Acute trauma is usually secondary to falls or other impact. This pathology is common in competitive and recreational runners.
Manifestations	Typical clinical manifestations of this pathology include lateral proximal thigh pain with radiation down the lateral thigh. There may be tenderness with proximal palpation. Pain persists during gait, ADL, and bed mobility activities.
Medical Management	Diagnosis is typically made by physical examination. Medical management includes rest and the use of oral NSAIDS. In more severe cases, corticosteroid injection may be used. Referral to physical therapy for continued management is important.
Physical Therapy Goals	Physical therapy goals include management of inflammation and pain and the restoration or maintenance of soft-tissue length, particularly the iliotibial band/tensor fascia lata complex.
Effective PT Interventions	The preferred treatment position is sidelying with the affected limb uphill.
	Cryotherapy is effective in controlling inflammation. Treatment sessions often can begin and end with cryotherapy techniques directly over the bursa region.

Trochanteric Bursitis, cont.

Continuous wave ultrasound over the distal two thirds of the ITB in preparation for stretching may be effective. Given the relatively large treatment area, an extended ultrasound treatment time is preferable.

Passive stretching of the ITB (hip adduction and extension in sidelying), though perhaps initially painful, increases length and decreases potential bursa irritation. Strengthening of abductors and general hip musculature may help alleviate precipitating factors.

Precautions   Cautious use of vigorous exercise or closed chain exercise until inflammation is well controlled is advisable.

References

American Society for Surgery of the Hand. (2001). Carpal tunnel syndrome. Retrieved October 15, 2005, from www.assh.org/Content/NavigationMenu/Patients_and_Public/Carpal_Tunnel_Syndrome/Carpal_Tunnel_Syndrome.htm.

Dutton, M. (2004). *Orthopedic examination, evaluation and intervention*. Philadelphia: McGraw Hill.

Goodman, C., Boissonault, W., & Fuller, K. (2003). *Pathology: Implications for the physical therapist*. Philadelphia: Saunders.

Gould, B. (2002). *Pathophysiology of health professions*. Philadelphia: Saunders.

Kisner, C., & Colby, L. (2002). *Therapeutic exercise foundations and techniques*. Philadelphia: F.A. Davis.

Lesh, S. (2000). *Clinical orthopedics for the physical therapist assistant*. Philadelphia: F.A. Davis.

McAfee, P. (2002). *Bracing treatment for idiopathic scoliosis*. Retrieved November 29, 2005, from www.spine-health.com/topics/cd/scoliosis/scoliosis.html.

Mckenzie, R.A. (1981). *The lumbar spine: Mechanical diagnosis and therapy*. Wellington, New Zealand: Spinal Publications.

Michael J. Fox Foundation for Parkinson's Research. (2005). *About Parkinson's*. Retrieved October 20, 2005, from www.michaeljfox.org/parkinsons/index.php.

Moore, K. (1985). *Clinically oriented anatomy*. Baltimore: Williams & Wilkins.

National Institute of Neurological Disorders and Strokes. (2005). *NINDS thoracic outlet syndrome information page*. Retrieved October 25, 2005, from www.ninds.nih.gov/disorders/thoracic/thoracic.htm.

National Multiple Sclerosis Society. (2005). *About MS*. Retrieved November 29, 2005, from www.nationalmssociety.org/about%20ms.asp.

Schapiro, R. (1999). *Symptoms management in multiple sclerosis*. New York: Demos.

Listing of Common Abbreviations

♀ —female
♂ —male
1—primary
2—secondary
a—before
ABG—arterial blood gas
ACL—anterior cruciate ligament
AD—Alzheimer disease
ADL—activities of daily living
AK—above knee
ALS—amyotrophic lateral sclerosis
AML—acute myelogenous leukemia
ANS—autonomic nervous system
ant.—anterior
AP—anteroposterior
ASCVD—arteriosclerotic cardiovascular disease
ASHD—arteriosclerotic heart disease
assist—assistance
B—bilateral, both
bid—twice a day
BK—below knee
BLE—both lower extremities
BPH—benign prostatic hypertrophy
BPM—beats per minute
BRP—bathroom privileges

BUN—blood urea nitrogen
BX, bx—biopsy
c—with
CA—cardiac arrest
Ca—cancer
CABG—coronary artery bypass graft
CAD—coronary artery disease
cath—catherization, catheter
CBC—complete blood count
CCs—chief complaints
CD—cardiovascular disease
CDH—congenital dislocation of hip
CF—cystic fibrosis
CHD—coronary heart disease
CHF—congestive heart failure
c/o—complaints of
COPD—chronic obstructive pulmonary disease
CP—cerebral palsy
CPM—continuous passive motion
CPR—cardiopulmonary resuscitation
CRF—chronic renal failure
CSF—cerebrospinal fluid
CVA—cerebrovascular accident
dc, DC—discontinue, discharge
d/c—discharge
DF—dorsiflexion
DJD—degenerative joint disease
DM—diabetes mellitus
DNR—do not resuscitate
DOB—date of birth
DOE—dypnea on exertion
DTR—deep tendon reflex
DVT—deep vein thrombosis
Dx—diagnosis
ECG (EKG)—electrocardiogram
EEG—electroencephalogram

EMG—electromyography

ER—emergency room, external rotation

E-Stim—electrical stimulation

Ev, ev—eversion

eval—evaluation

ex.—exercise

ext.—extension

FES—functional electrical stimulation

flex—flexion

F/U—follow up

FWB—full weight bearing

FWW, fw/w—front wheeled walker

fx—fracture

GMT—gross motor test

Gt.—gait

H&P—history and physical examination

HAV—hepatitis A virus

Hb, hgb—hemoglobin

HBV—hepatitis B virus

HCFA—health care financing administration

HCT, Hct—hematocrit

HCV—hepatitis C virus

HD—hemodialysis, hip disarticulation, hearing distance

HDV—hepatitis D virus

HEV—hepatitis E virus

HEP –home exercise program

HF—heart failure

HHA—home health aide

HNP—herniated nucleus pulposus

h/o—history of

HP—hot pack

HPI—history of present illness

Hr—hour

HS—hamstrings

Hx—history

I—independent(ly)

I & D—incision and drainage

ICP—intracranial pressure, intermittent compression pump

IDDM—insulin-dependent diabetes mellitus

IEP—individual education program

int.—internal

IV—intravenous, inversion

KD—knee disarticulation

L—left

LAQ—long arc quadriceps

LAT, lat—lateral

LBP—low back pain

LE—lower extremity

LLL—left lower lobe (of lung)

LMN—lower motor neuron

LOB—loss of balance

MH—moist heat

MI—myocardial infarction

min—minutes

min.—minimal, minimum

mm(s)—manual muscle test

MS—mental status, mitral stenosis, musculoskeletal, multiple sclerosis

N/A—not able

NAD—no apparent distress

n & v—nausea and vomiting

NIDDM—noninsulin dependent diabetes mellitus

noc.—night

NPO, npo—nothing by mouth

NSAIDS—nonsteroidal anti-inflammatory drugs

NSR—normal sinus rhythm

NWB—nonweight bearing

N/V/D—nausea, vomiting, diarrhea

occ—occasional

OOB—out of bed

p—after, post

p—pulse

pc—after meals

PCL—posterior cruciate ligament
per—by
PMH—past medical history
po—by mouth
POC—plan of care
post—posterior
post op—postoperative
pps—pulse per second
PRE—progressive resistive exercise
pre op—preoperative
PRN, prn—as needed
PROM—passive range of motion
pt.—patient
PWB—partial weight bearing
q2h—every 2 hours
Qam, qm—every morning
qd—every day
qh—every hour
q_h—every hour
qid—four times a day
qod—every other day
qpm, qn—every night
R—right
R—respiration
RA—rheumatoid arthritis
RBC, rbc—red blood cell, red blood count
RD—respiratory distress
RDS—respiratory distress syndrome
re:—regarding
re-ed—reeducation
reps—repetitions
RL—right lateral
RLE—right lower extremity
R/O, r/o—rule out
ROM—range of motion
rot.—rotation

RUE—right upper extremity
RUQ—right upper quadrant
RV—residual volume, right ventricle
Rx—drug, prescription, therapy
SAQ—short arc quadriceps
SBA—stand-by assist
SCI—spinal cord injury
SD—shoulder disarticulation
sec—second
SLR—straight-leg raise
SOB—shortness of breath
stat—immediately
STG—short-term goal
str.—strength
Sx—symptoms
TDD—tentative discharge data
TDP—tentative discharge plan
T.E.D.'s—antiembolism stockings
TFs—transfers
THA—total hip arthroplasty
THR—total hip replacement
TIA—transient ischemic attack
tid—three times a day
TKA—total knee arthroplasty
TKE—total knee extension
TKR—total knee replacement
TLC—total lung capacity
TPR—temperature, pulse, respiration
trng.—training
TTWB—toe touch weight bearing
TWB—touch weight bearing
tx—treatment, traction
UE—upper extremity
U & L, U/L—upper and lower
UMN—upper motor neuron
URI—upper respiratory infection

UTI—urinary tract infection
US—ultrasound
VC—vital capacity
VS—vital signs
VT—ventricular tachycardia
WBC, wbc—white blood cell, white blood count
WC, w/c—wheelchair
w/cm²—watts per square centimeter
WFL—within functional limits
w/p—whirlpool
w/o—without
WNL—within normal limits
X—times
YO—year(s) old

References

Cohen, B.J. (2004). *Medical terminology: An illustrated guide*.
   Baltimore: Lippincott Williams & Wilkins.

Gylys, B.A., & Wedding, M.E. (2005). *Medical terminology systems: A body systems approach*. Philadelphia: F.A. Davis.

Lukan, M. (2001). *Documentation for physical therapist assistants*.
   Philadelphia: F.A. Davis.

Index

W

Y

Z